Digital Media and Participatory Cultures of Health and Illness

This book explores how the complex scenario of platforms, practices and content in the contemporary digital landscape is shaping participatory cultures of health and illness.

The everyday use of digital and social media platforms has major implications for the production, seeking and sharing of health information, and raises important questions about health peer support, power relations, trust, privacy and knowledge. To address these questions, this book navigates contemporary forms of participation that develop through mundane digital practices, like tweeting about the latest pandemic news or keeping track of our daily runs with Fitbit or Strava. In doing so, it explores both radical activist practices and more ordinary forms of participation that can gradually lead to social and/or cultural changes in how we understand and experience health and illness. While drawing upon digital media studies and the sociology of health and illness, this book offers theoretical and methodological insights from a decade of empirical research of health-related digital practices that span from digital health advocacy to illness-focused social media uses.

Accessible and engaging, this book is ideal for scholars and students interested in digital media, digital activism, health advocacy and digital health.

Stefania Vicari is Senior Lecturer in Digital Sociology at the University of Sheffield, UK. Her research interests include the general areas of digital participation, digital health and digital methods. Her works have appeared in a number of journals including *Information, Communication and Society*; *Media, Culture and Society*; *New Media and Society; Social Media + Society*; *Social Movement Studies* and *Current Sociology*.

Routledge Studies in New Media and Cyberculture

Digital Media, Sharing and Everyday Life
Jenny Kennedy

Digital Icons
Memes, Martyrs and Avatars
Yasmin Ibrahim

Artificial Intelligence in Cultural Production
Critical Perspectives on Digital Platforms
Dal Yong Jin

Loving Fanfiction
Exploring the Role of Emotion in Online Fandoms
Brit Kelley

Posthuman Capitalism
Dancing with Data in the Digital Economy
Yasmin Ibrahim

Smartphone Communication
Interactions in the App Ecosystem
Francisco Yus

Upgrade Culture and Technological Change
The Business of the Future
Adam Richard Rottinghaus

Digital Media and Participatory Cultures of Health and Illness
Stefania Vicari

For more information about this series, please visit: https://www.routledge.com/Routledge-Studies-in-New-Media-and-Cyberculture/book-series/RSINC

Digital Media and Participatory Cultures of Health and Illness

Stefania Vicari

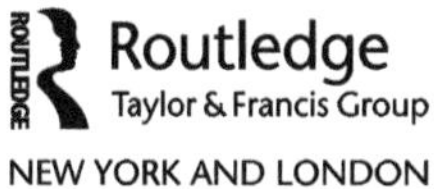

NEW YORK AND LONDON

First published 2022
by Routledge
605 Third Avenue, New York, NY 10158

and by Routledge
2 Park Square, Milton Park, Abingdon, Oxon, OX14 4RN

Routledge is an imprint of the Taylor & Francis Group, an Informa business

Library of Congress Cataloging-in-Publication Data
Names: Vicari, Stefania, author.
Title: Digital media and participatory cultures of health and illness / Stefania Vicari.
Description: New York, NY : Routledge, [2022] | Series: Routledge studies in new media and cyberculture | Includes bibliographical references and index.
Subjects: LCSH: Health promotion—Technological innovations. | Digital media.
Classification: LCC RA427.8 .V53 2022 (print) | LCC RA427.8 (ebook) | DDC 362.10285—dc23/eng/20211013
LC record available at https://lccn.loc.gov/2021033716
LC ebook record available at https://lccn.loc.gov/2021033717

ISBN: 978-1-138-60312-7 (hbk)
ISBN: 978-1-032-16958-3 (pbk)
ISBN: 978-0-429-46914-5 (ebk)

DOI: 10.4324/9780429469145

Typeset in Times New Roman
by Apex CoVantage, LLC

Contents

List of Figures and Tables vi
Acknowledgements viii

1 Introduction: Pandemic Snapshots, Digital Media and Participatory Cultures of Health and Illness 1

PART 1: Theoretical Foundations 13

2 Digital Media, Participation and Citizenship 15
3 Health Advocacy and Activism 38

PART 2: Digitised and Networked Health 59

4 The Rise of the "Epatient" in the Internet That Was 61
5 From Patient Organisations to Patient Networks 75

PART 3: Platforms 97

6 Participatory Cultures of Health and Illness on Mainstream Social Media 99
7 Participatory Cultures of Health and Illness on Digital Health Platforms 133

8 Conclusion: Understanding Participatory Cultures of Health and Illness in Contemporary Societies 153

Index 159

Figures and Tables

Figures

1.1 BBC News tweet about Guo Jing's diary. 2
1.2 Three Twitter-selected "Top tweets" mentioning "Steve Walsh" in the morning of 11 February 2020. 3
1.3 First #LongCovid tweet. 4
1.4 Samantha Batt-Rawden and the "yellow army" on Twitter. 6
4.1 "Telemedicine", "eHealth" and "mHealth" on PubMed 1980-present. 62
5.1 Digital Mechanisms on the websites of rare disease patient organisations. 88
6.1 Storytelling tweet (1) (anonymised and paraphrased). 113
6.2 Storytelling tweet (2). 114
6.3 Storytelling tweet (3). 114
6.4 Storytelling tweet (4) (anonymised and paraphrased). 115
6.5 Storytelling tweet (5). 115
6.6 Storytelling tweet (6) (anonymised and paraphrased). 116
6.7 Non-storytelling tweet (1). 117
6.8 Non-storytelling tweet (2). 117
6.9 Button sharing generating the pre-modified version of the tweet of Figure 6.8. 118
6.10 Non-storytelling tweet (3) (anonymised and paraphrased). 118
6.11 Issue publics, communities of practice and epistemic communities on social media. 120
6.12 Sources of information in storytelling and non-storytelling tweets. 121
6.13 National Hereditary Breast Cancer Helpline announcing the passing of Louise Mallendar on Facebook. 123

Tables

5.1 Rare disease and patients' advocacy organisations. 77
5.2 The identity of rare disease patients' advocacy organisations. 79

5.3 The areas of action of rare disease patients' advocacy organisations. 81
5.4 A typology of rare disease patients' advocacy organisations. 85
5.5 Top linked to websites. 90
6.1 Top broadcasters of BRCA content in the 2013 sample period. 103
6.2 Top gatekeepers of BRCA content in the 2013 sample period. 103
6.3 Top broadcasters of BRCA content in the 2015 sample period. 105
6.4 Top gatekeepers of BRCA content in the 2015 sample period. 106
6.5 Hashtag pairs with top 10 frequencies over the 2013 sample period. 108
6.6 Hashtag pairs with top 10 frequencies over the 2015 sample period. 110
6.7 Personal storytelling and communication practices in the 2017 sample period. 112
6.8 Top 4 users quoting scientific sources or medical news in the 2017 sample period. 124

Acknowledgements

My daughter Noa tells me that this book could never be as long as a Harry Potter one. She is right. And yet, it draws upon projects, thoughts, conversations and events that cover the past ten years of my life.

Chapters 5 and 6 present research that was funded by two grants from the Wellcome Trust and I am grateful to the anonymous reviewers of *Information, Communication and Society*, *Social Media + Society* and *New Media and Society* and to members of the Seminar on the Analysis of Social Processes and Structures at Sorbonne University who provided feedback on previous outputs based on this research.

I am also thankful to mentors, colleagues and friends from my time at Emory, Sassari, Leicester and Sheffield who, in the most different ways, have inspired and supported me through the thinking and making of this book: Roberto Franzosi, Gianluca de Fazio, Laura Iannelli, Anders Hansen, Grazia De Michele, Paul Reilly, Helen Kennedy, Maria Francesca Murru, and Suay Özkula. Thanks also to students in my modules *Protest and publics in the network society* and *Digital media and social change*, who prompted me to reflect on meanings and understandings of digital media and participation across cultures and places.

My father is the reason I started thinking about health and illness years ago. My mum and my brother a good part of the reason I kept thinking about it. So, this book is a little bit about them too.

Finally, I thank Noa, Anna, and Franco. Noa, for her thoughts. Anna, for her smiles. Franco, for all the rest that matters.

1 Introduction

Pandemic Snapshots, Digital Media and Participatory Cultures of Health and Illness

Five Pandemic Snapshots

Snapshot 1: "Social Media Diarists" and "Digital Whistleblowers"

It was January 2020 when Guo Jing's diary from quarantined Wuhan made it to BBC News (see Figure 1.1). Jing wrote from the first epicentre of the Covid-19 pandemic. Through cautious tinkering with Chinese social media (Yang, 2020), she narrated the first lockdown, often offering critical reflections about the handling of the pandemic outbreak by the local and national authorities (BBC News, 2020a).

A social worker and feminist activist, Jing was one of the few who provided narrative accounts of what was happening in Wuhan. Possibly due to her combining personal storytelling with critiques of the social injustice she witnessed in the locked down city, some of her diary entries became viral in the Chinese social media ecosystem, receiving over 100,000 views. Her posts would often end with a call to "connect":

> I would like to become a connector. I hope to build connections with more and more people. So we can act together. My WeChat[1] ID is: 1461177244. If you are in Wuhan and would like to be a volunteer, please message me offline and let me know, so we can do something together.
>
> (Yang, 2020)

Guo Jing and other "social media diarists" followed the "digital whistleblowers" (Yang, 2020) who had first posted about a SARS-like illness in their WeChat groups at the end of December 2019, when the Chinese public health authorities were still silencing information related to it (BBC News, 2020b). While these citizens' original intention was merely to alert friends of potential health risks, their messages were cross-posted on different social media platforms and reached a wider audience than originally intended. This allegedly caught the eye of Chinese public security authorities, who questioned and punished these citizens for sharing critical information. Media and communication scholar Guobin Yang (2021) suggests that pandemic diaries and

DOI: 10.4324/9780429469145-1

BBC News (UK)
@BBCNews
Coronavirus Wuhan diary: Living alone in a city gone quiet
BBC NEWS
Coronavirus Wuhan diary: Living alone in a city gone quiet
Loneliness, emptiness, and hyper-hygiene - one woman describes life in a city gone quiet.
bbc.com
6:03 AM · Jan 30, 2020 · SocialFlow
45 Retweets 5 Quote Tweets 101 Likes

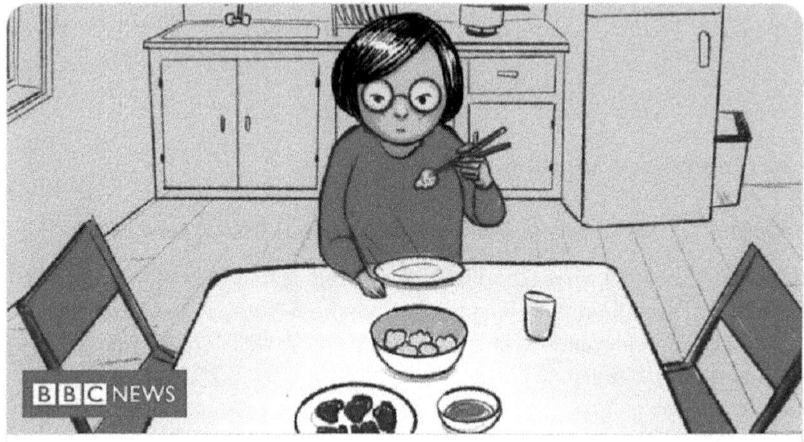

Figure 1.1 BBC News tweet about Guo Jing's diary.

whistleblowing were a form of "endurance art": they produced meanings that reached far beyond their original purpose and context. But what agency did this meaning acquire while navigating across a range of digital platforms? Was writing and sharing at that time, in that place and on those very platforms, a participatory act?

Snapshot 2: Stephanie, Jack and Imran

In February 2020 the daily updates about what was to become the Covid-19 pandemic were starting to look grim in the Western side of the world. If you were in the UK, you probably found yourself learning about

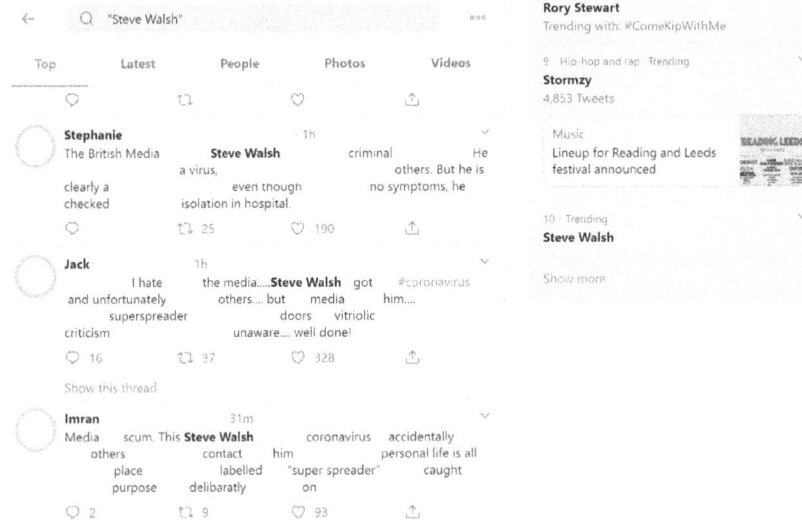

Figure 1.2 Three Twitter-selected "Top tweets" mentioning "Steve Walsh" in the morning of 11 February 2020.

"super-spreaders"—individuals who "transmit infections to far more people than the majority do" (Boseley, 2020). On 11 February, "Steve Walsh", the name of the first "super-spreader" identified in the UK, was trending on the UK Twitter (see Figure 1.2).

On that day, Stephanie, Jack and Imran[2] were tweeting about Steve Walsh and targeting "the media", complaining about the way the news about contagion was being handled. In fact, during the previous two days, the "legacy" media Stephanie, Jack and Imran referred to (e.g., BBC, The Guardian, The Telegraph) had been feeding us details about Steve Walsh's January trip to Singapore, where the virus was passed on to him. Further transmission, we were told, happened during Walsh's stop-over in France and then again in the UK, when he finally made it home on the 28th of January (Siddique, 2020). When, back in 2003, similar events were happening in relation to the first Severe Acute Respiratory Syndrome (SARS CoV) outbreak, we would not have been surprised to hear similar grievances in private conversations with friends or relatives or read them in formal complaints to media regulators. But what difference does it make that they are now also finding a platform on Twitter?

Snapshot 3: We Are Long Covid

In the spring of 2020, Elisa Perego, an Italian archaeologist, was struggling with the cyclical effects of a Covid-19 infection. Perego's symptoms and disease progression differed from the pathway discussed in the then-available scientific papers. When on 20 May 2020 Perego tweeted of her "#LongCovid" (see Figure 1.3), probably little did she know that in a matter of a few months "Long Covid" would become a WHO-endorsed label to define the condition of people living with the long-term effects of a Covid-19 infection (Perego et al., 2020).

Neither would she have imagined that an editorial in Nature and a piece in the Social Science & Medicine journal would call for patients to get involved in defining what Long Covid is and what symptoms make for this condition (Callard & Perego, 2021; Fox, 2020; Nature, 2020). As a matter of fact, following Perego's tweet, the term "Long Covid" came to be adopted by an increasing number of patient groups discussing symptoms primarily on online platforms, to the point that the term was soon also interjected by the legacy media and gradually adopted in official scientific contexts and policy documents. By August 2020, "Long Covid" had turned into a scientific label, meaning that from the domain of folksonomies it had transferred into that of formalised taxonomies.

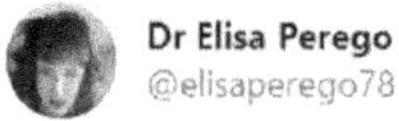

L'infettivologo: "Il 20% dei malati resta positivo al virus per 40 giorni"
Paul Garner, professore di malattie infettive alla Liverpool School of Tropical Medicine, a sette settimane dal primo tampone è ancora positivo. E non è un ...
rep.repubblica.it
7:17 pm · 20 May 2020 · Twitter for Android

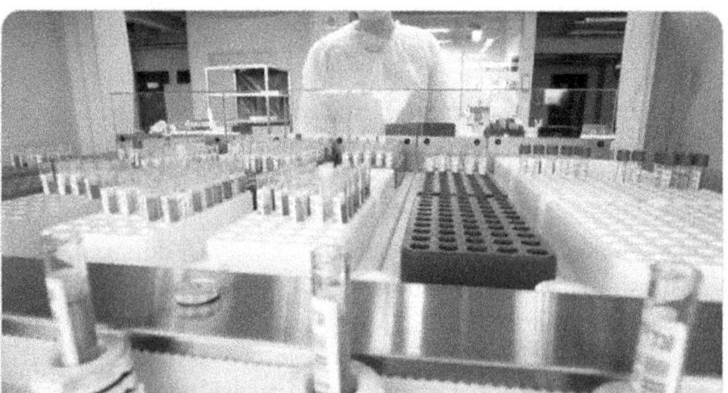

Figure 1.3 First #LongCovid tweet.

Words do matter. Using "Long Covid" rather than "Post Covid", for instance, dramatically changes the ontology of the condition: it acknowledges the relevance and impact of morbidity in the life of those who have "mild" infections or have "recovered" from hospitalisation, it potentially challenges response strategies only primarily focused on "saving lives", it legitimises the voices of those who experience symptoms that are not (yet) officially recorded and it redraws attention to the risk for every member of the population, including those perceived as safer (e.g., children and people without "underlying conditions").

Long Covid is certainly not the first illness label created through patients finding each other online but it did move "from patients, through various media, to formal clinical and policy channels in just a few months . . . and demonstrates how patients marshalled epistemic authority" (Callard & Perego, 2021, p. 1). But then, what does the Long Covid story tell us about the value of patient knowledge and expertise for how health and illness are conceptualised, researched, treated, lived, policed, and politicised in contemporary societies?

Snapshot 4: Tracking, Tracing and Being Responsible. Right, But What About My Data?

By June 2020, the debate about the way technology could enhance public response to the Covid-19 crisis was in full swing. The question surfacing in the months up to June was whether and how apps could be used to support symptom tracking, contact tracing and immunity certification, with a range of societal, political, legal and ethical perspectives animating the debate (Ada Lovelace Institute, 2020a). The very controversy, at that point, centred on how contact tracing should work. Contact tracing was thought to provide an early warning to people who have been in contact with someone who is or may be infected with Covid-19. The warning enables individuals to take action and *responsibly* prevent spreading the virus onwards, by, for instance, self-isolating.

The issue was not so much on the usefulness of automated systems of contact tracing but rather on how data should be collected and stored in the process. In practice, privacy soon became the key object of the debate. There were broadly two main options to be considered: "centralised" or "decentralised" systems (Fraser et al., 2020). In the centralised architecture, when an individual is diagnosed with infection, their contact history, in the form of phone IDs, gets uploaded to a server that then sends notifications to the relevant contacts. In the decentralised architecture, infection data and notifications are instead sent over the phone network. Decentralised systems only use a server for updating tracing rules and collecting summary statistics. The question then often centred on whether it was ethically acceptable for personal data to be centrally stored and whether this solution would gain public trust, and hence a successful app uptake.

With the UK deciding to drop its plans to adopt a centralised system (Kelion, 2020), the decentralised digital contact tracing architecture became the dominant paradigm globally (Ada Lovelace Institute, 2020b). As Google and Apple provide the operating system running on most smartphones, switching to the decentralised architecture meant, in practice, developing a contact tracing system based on their services and protocols, with Google and Apple's exposure notification API (Application Processing Interface) becoming the gateway to achieve contact tracing. And yet, does it matter at all that two giant corporations became the means to develop an essential element of public health response strategies around the world?

Snapshot 5. Blue Hearts Defeat the Yellow Army

On 29 December 2020, Samantha Batt-Rawden noticed that her Twitter feed was getting populated by an increasing number of accounts whose handles were marked by smiley emojis (see Figure 1.4).

An UK intensive care doctor and the founder of the Doctors' Association UK, Batt-Rawden had been advocating for the UK National Health Service (NHS) since the early stages of the pandemic, often questioning the UK Government's claims that the NHS was fully prepared to face a public crisis and highlighting its

Thread
Dr Samantha Batt-Rawden
@sbattrawden
I feel I have missed something crucial, wtf is up with people putting smiley faces on their profile and why are they mask-hating/anti-lockdown/opposite of smiley?
3:45 pm · 29 Dec 2020 · Twitter for iPhone
34 Retweets 4 Quote Tweets 493 Likes
Tweet your reply
Reply
Dr Samantha Batt-Rawden @sbattrawden · 29 Dec 2020
Replying to @sbattrawden
What I have I done. I seem to have provoked a bright yellow army. Welp.
39
6
144

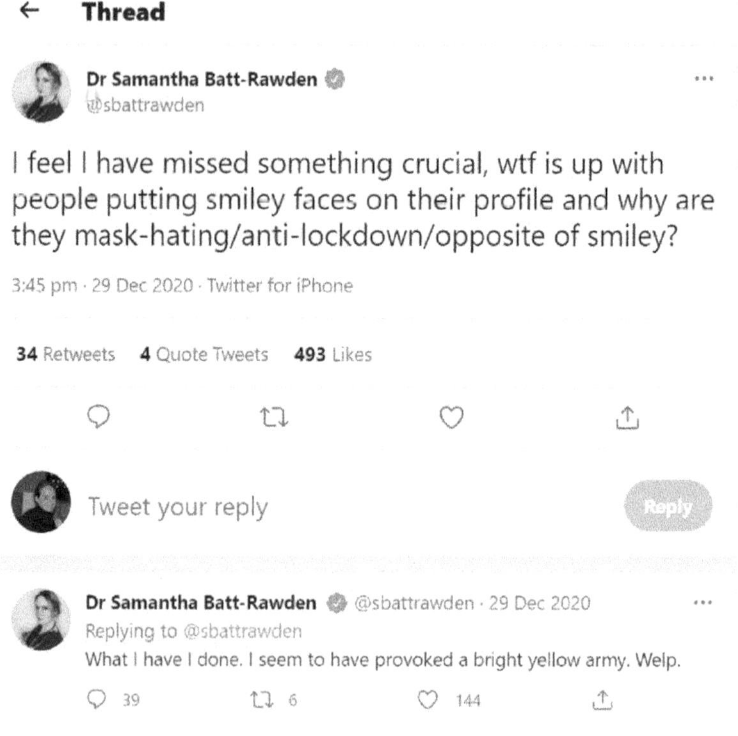

Figure 1.4 Samantha Batt-Rawden and the "yellow army" on Twitter.

lack of support for those working on the frontline (Batt-Rawden, 2020; Campbell, 2020). Through the early stages of the Covid-19 emergency, Batt-Rawden gradually became a visible actor of the pandemic in the UK, both growing social media influence, especially on Twitter, and sourcing legacy media content through opinion pieces for the daily press (e.g., The Guardian, The Independent) and appearances in TV News programmes (e.g., Good Morning Britain).

The "bright yellow army" Batt-Rawden was noticing in late December 2020 was a very heterogeneous group of Covid-19 sceptical accounts broadly advocating against lockdown restrictions, mask wearing and "bad science". These accounts' focus on science and data is perhaps unsurprising, given that existing research shows that Covid-19 scepticism is often itself data-driven, grounded in critiques about the sources of data and data visualizations used to justify public policies (Lee et al., 2021). Some of the smiley accounts' bios linked to the webpage of the "#smilesmatter movement" (smilesmatter, 2021), which at the time of writing still offers an entire section on "Why It's Time To Reject Bad Science On Covid Restrictions". Other smiley accounts linked to the website of PANDA:

> A group of multi-disciplinary professionals, who perceived the global reaction to Covid, and lockdown in particular, as overwrought and damaging to the point of causing a great tear in the fabric of society. . . . PANDA stands for open science and rational debate, for replacing flawed science with good science and for retrieving liberty and prosperity from the clutches of a dystopian "new normal".
>
> (PANDA, 2021)

Most likely in response to the increasing visibility of these accounts on Twitter and, more generally, to counter the wave of offensive messages that herself and other UK medical doctors and nurses were receiving on the platform, in early January 2021 Batt-Rawden launched the #NHSBlueheart campaign, asking people to add a blue heart emoji next to their Twitter handle to show their support for the NHS (Molyneaux, 2021). Blue hearts instantly flooded UK Twitter, outnumbering the yellow army in a matter of hours. Does this story suggest that emojis and hashtags somehow matter when it comes to participation, civil liberties, science, data and health policing? And if so, how, to whom and for how long do they matter?

A Book About Digital Media and Participatory Cultures of Health and Illness

This book is not about Covid-19, though it was written through it. Each and every one of the snapshots discussed above, however, touches upon at least one of the core issues that make this book what it is: a view into the way digital media are now central to how we live, experience, understand, and construct our personal and collective relationships with health and illness.

This book is about "participation" (Carpentier, 2011; Iannelli, 2016) because it explores how the centrality mentioned above shapes opportunities for citizens to craft and voice their opinions, experiences, interactions and forms of resistance connected to health and illness. Needless to say, the political, economic and technological structures of the digital ecosystem, along with its cultural environment, have a strong impact on how this participation takes shape through the production of meaning and its impact on decision-making. In exploring the way citizens participate in defining health and illness, this book sees participation through the lens of power, namely exploring how the contemporary digital maintains or disrupts pre-existing structures of power. Power dynamics emerge in relation to, for instance, health policy or research decision-making (see Chapter 4), knowledge production (see Chapter 5), expertise (see Chapter 6), and self-care (Chapter 7).

This book is about "participatory cultures" because it navigates contemporary forms of digitally enhanced participation as embedded in mundane practices, that is, ordinary aspects of our everyday life (Jenkins et al., 2016). In so doing, it explores both digital activist practices (Lievrouw, 2011, p. 19) explicitly meant to challenge accepted or traditional ways to see health and illness in relation to society, culture, and politics and more ordinary forms of digital engagement that may ultimately lead to social and/or cultural change in traditional understandings and practices related to health and illness.

This book is about "health and illness" because despite health having a strong personal and "embodied" dimension (Brown et al., 2004), health access and care are among the most regulated, policed and often politicized, hence contested, issues in contemporary societies. 1990s and early 2000s research (e.g., Brown & Zavestoski, 2004; Epstein, 1996) has clearly pointed to the emergence of different and more or less institutionalised forms of resistance to accepted ways of understanding and regulating health access, care and research. In most cases, these instances have been shown to advocate for widened participation in the domain of health and illness, carving space for patients' and carers' voices to participate in self-care decision-making, scientific development, health care policing and drug approval systems. And yet, still little do we know about how contemporary digital ecosystems shape these dynamics (Lupton, 2017), with research just starting to explore how extremely heterogeneous forms of participation are unravelling through the digital (see, for example, Petersen et al., 2019; Petrakaki et al., 2021; Vicari & Cappai. 2016). To contribute to and advance this discussion, this book brings together Digital media research, the Sociology of health and illness and Science and Technologies Studies.

Overview of the Book

Tentative answers to the questions advanced at the end of each pandemic snapshot presented above are hidden in the pages to follow and come together in the concluding chapter. The book develops through three main parts. First, it navigates foundational theories, concepts and debates that become relevant when we think of how digital media are woven into contemporary cultures of health and illness. In particular, Chapter 2, "Digital media, participation, and citizenship", provides a conceptual introduction for interpreting participatory dynamics in increasingly digitised societies. It does so, first of all, by focusing on the context in which contemporary digital media platforms have progressively emerged and developed. It discusses shifts in the Western media ecosystem, particularly in the way media content is produced, consumed and used and how these changes have gradually shaped participatory practices. This discussion introduces and engages with concepts that have emerged as central to contemporary digital media research: produsage, platformisation and datafication. The chapter then progresses by arguing that these shifts have enhanced the surfacing of specific discursive practices, with public sphere dynamics, counterpublics and networked publics emerging through new user-generated curation practices and visual cultures.

Chapter 3, "Health advocacy and activism", continues the conceptual journey started in Chapter 1 but focuses on pre-digital participatory practices emerging in relation to health and illness. The chapter begins by exploring contemporary definitions of health advocacy and activism and discussing the way these have seen the progressive emergence of patient organisations and groups lobbying for the direct participation of patients in health policy and research decision-making. The chapter engages with debates about the so-called "scientisation" of policy decision-making, which argue for or against the view that scientific evidence should be the primary voice to inform policy making. The chapter explores specific examples of patient activism like the French AIDS and autistic movements and follows their development since the 1980s. The second part of the chapter redirects the focus to a number of concepts that are key to the discussion of health activist and advocacy action and are closely interrelated: illness identity, illness narrative, self-advocacy, experiential knowledge and lay expertise. Finally, the chapter engages with these concepts to explore the advocacy action promoted by patient communities focusing on hereditary conditions in general and rare disease patient communities in particular.

The second part of the book starts linking together health, illness, and the digital, by focusing on early examples and conceptualisations of digitised and networked health. Chapter 4, "The rise of the epatient in the Internet that was", while focusing on early digital media practices, presents two key conceptualisations of information and communication technologies in relation to health and illness: the "service delivery" and the "epatient" paradigms. These paradigms show how early digital platforms and spaces have often been framed as functional to enhance individuals' experiences of health and illness. The first part of the chapter focuses on the "service delivery" paradigm, according to which technology in general and information and communication technologies in particular are means to improve the delivery of services from producers to consumers. The second part of the chapter focuses on the "epatient paradigm", according to which online platforms participate in processes that see patients as more directly engaged with their self-care and with the care of others, individually and collectively.

Chapter 5, "From patient organisations to patient networks", explores the relationship between digital media and contemporary health advocacy by navigating the affordances of digital media and communication for advocacy organisations representing patient communities. The chapter draws on an empirical piece of work carried out by Vicari and Cappai (2016) that specifically focused on rare disease patient organisations. The first part explores the role of organisation websites in defining the identity and the remit of action of rare disease patient advocacy. The second part of the chapter argues that digital mechanisms (i.e., technological elements embedded in or connected to organisation websites) enhance health knowledge co-production, individualised means of public engagement and alternative informational pathways, ultimately bolstering the development of health-centred networked publics.

The third and final part of the book is entirely centred on the role of contemporary digital platforms in hindering or enhancing specific participatory practices related to health and illness. Chapter 6, "Participatory cultures of health and illness on mainstream social media", explores health issue publics forming on mainstream social media. It does so by drawing upon empirical work that I conducted in 2017 and 2020 to explore hereditary cancer communities on Twitter. Needless to say, choosing one platform among many means failing to provide a comprehensive discussion of the social media ecology characterising contemporary societies. The chapter's focus on Twitter, however, allows one to explore the potential emergence of health-centred participatory practices in contexts that are extremely different to the more dedicated and often contained digital spaces addressed in early Internet studies and partially replicated in similarly contained spaces on contemporary social media platforms (e.g., Facebook groups). The chapter explores four dynamics in specific terms: curation, framing, storytelling and epistemic work and concludes by reflecting on the complex relationship between mainstream social media platforms and contemporary cultures of health and illness.

Chapter 7, "Participatory cultures of health and illness on digital health platforms", draws attention to platforms designed and used primarily to monitor, store, track, and/or record health-related personal information. First, it engages with studies focused on the political economy and the technological infrastructure of these platforms. In so doing, it explores a number of aspects hindering bottom-up practices able to overcome both the ephemeral rhetoric of "participation" often used by corporate platform providers and the technological constraints inherently inscribed in platformed systems. The chapter then progresses by building on socio-cultural and material interpretations of digital health practices to explore the agency exerted by platform users despite adverse political economic structures and constraining technologies. It does so by drawing attention to scholarly work interested in everyday digital health practices that domesticate technological devices, algorithmic systems, and data in their social, cultural, and material contexts.

Finally, Chapter 8, "Understanding participatory cultures of health and illness in contemporary societies", summarises the contribution of the book by advancing five arguments that address the questions raised at the beginning of the present chapter. It does so by focusing on digital participation as connective, personalised and crowdsourced agency; the media side of digital participation; lay expertise as a digital participatory practice; digital participation through, or despite, corporate gateways (aka, the usual foes); and digital participation as platformed. Ultimately, these points offer concluding reflections on why and how "the digital" matters when it comes to understanding participatory cultures of health and illness in contemporary societies.

Notes

1. WeChat (or Wēixìn) is a Chinese multipurpose social media platform that provides mobile instant messaging services similar to those of its Western counterpart WhatsApp (Lien & Cao, 2014).
2. Twitter handles and post content in Figure 1.2 have been edited for ethical reasons.

Reference List

#smilesmatter (2021). *Why it's time to reject bad science on Covid restrictions*. https://smilesmatter.info/why-its-time-to-reject-bad-science-on-covid/. Retrieved 17 June 2021.

Ada Lovelace Institute (2020a, April 20). *Exit through the app store?* www.adalovelaceinstitute.org/wp-content/uploads/2020/04/Ada-Lovelace-Institute-Rapid-Evidence-Review-Exit-through-the-App-Store-April-2020-2.pdf

Ada Lovelace Institute (2020b, July 9). *COVID-19 digital contact tracing tracker*. www.adalovelaceinstitute.org/project/covid-19-digital-contact-tracing-tracker/

Batt-Rawden, S. (2020, December 30). As a critical care doctor I'm scared of what the NHS is facing: The vaccine rollout can't come soon enough. *Independent*. www.independent.co.uk/voices/coronavirus-nhs-hospitals-doctors-nurses-covid-b1780398.html

BBC (2020a, February 7). Li Wenliang: Coronavirus kills Chinese whistleblower doctor. *BBC News*. www.bbc.co.uk/news/world-asia-china-51403795

BBC (2020b, January 30). Coronavirus Wuhan diary: Living alone in a city gone quiet. *BBC News*. www.bbc.co.uk/news/world-asia-china-51276656

Boseley, S. (2020, March 3). Super-spreaders: What are they and how are they transmitting coronavirus? *The Guardian*. www.theguardian.com/world/2020/feb/10/what-are-super-spreaders-coronavirus

Brown, P., & Zavestoski, S. (2004). Social movements in health: An introduction. *Sociology of Health & Illness*, *26*(6), 679–694.

Brown, P., Zavestoski, S., McCormick, S., Mayer, B., Morello-Frosch, R., & Gasior Altman, R. (2004). Embodied health movements: New approaches to social movements in health. *Sociology of Health & Illness*, *26*(1), 50–80.

Callard, F., & Perego, E. (2021). How and why patients made Long Covid. *Social Science & Medicine*, *268*, 113426.

Campbell, D. (2020, September 5). More than 1,000 UK doctors want to quit NHS over handling of pandemic. *The Guardian*. www.theguardian.com/society/2020/sep/05/more-than-1000-doctors-want-to-quit-nhs-over-handling-of-pandemic

Carpentier, N. (2011). *Media and participation: A site of ideological-democratic struggle*. Intellect.

Epstein, S. (1996). *Impure science: AIDS, activism, and the politics of knowledge* (Vol. 7). University of California Press.

Fox, S. (2020, November 11). *How connection can lead to change*. https://susannahfox.com/2020/11/11/how-connection-can-lead-to-change/

Fraser, C., Abeler-Dörner, L., Ferretti, L., Parker, M., Kendall, M., & Bonsall, D. (2020). *Digital contact tracing: Comparing the capabilities of centralised and decentralised data architectures to effectively suppress the COVID-19 epidemic whilst maximising freedom of movement and maintaining privacy*. University of Oxford. https://github.com/BDI-pathogens/covid-19_instant_tracing/blob/master/Centralised%20and%20decentralised%20systems%20for%20contact%20tracing.pdf.

Iannelli, L. (2016). *Hybrid politics: Media and participation*. Sage.

Jenkins, H., Ito, M., & boyd, d. (2016). *Participatory culture in a networked era: A conversation on youth, learning, commerce, and politics*. John Wiley & Sons.

Kelion, L. (2020, June 18). UK virus-tracing app switches to Apple-Google model. *BBC News*. www.bbc.co.uk/news/technology-53095336

Lee, C., Yang, T., Inchoco, G. D., Jones, G. M., & Satyanarayan, A. (2021, May). Viral visualizations: How coronavirus skeptics use orthodox data practices to promote unorthodox science online. In *Proceedings of the 2021 CHI Conference on Human Factors in Computing Systems* (pp. 1–18).

Lien, C. H., & Cao, Y. (2014). Examining WeChat users' motivations, trust, attitudes, and positive word-of-mouth: Evidence from China. *Computers in Human Behavior*, *41*, 104–111.

Lievrouw, L. (2011). *Alternative and activist new media*. John Wiley & Sons.

Lupton, D. (2017). Introduction. In Lupton, D. (Ed.) *Digitised health, medicine and risk* (pp. 1–3). Routledge.

Molyneaux, I. (2021, January 7). Why blue hearts are appearing next to people's names on Twitter. *My London*. www.mylondon.news/news/health/blue-hearts-appearing-next-peoples-19580263

Nature (2020). Long COVID: Let patients help define long-lasting COVID symptoms. *Nature*, *586*, 170.

PANDA (2021). *Who we are*. www.pandata.org/about/. Retrieved 17 June 2021.

Perego, E., Callard, F., Stras, L., Melville-Johannesson, B., Pope, R., & Alwan, N. (2020, October 1). Why we need to keep using the patient-made term "Long Covid". *BMJ Opinion*. https://blogs.bmj.com/bmj/2020/10/01/why-we-need-to-keep-using-the-patient-made-term-long-covid/

Petersen, A., Schermuly, A. C., & Anderson, A. (2019). The shifting politics of patient activism: From bio-sociality to bio-digital citizenship. *Health*, *23*(4), 478–494.

Petrakaki, D., Hilberg, E., & Waring, J. (2021). The cultivation of digital health citizenship. *Social Science & Medicine*, *270*, 113675.

Siddique, H. (2020, February 10). 'Super-spreader' brought coronavirus from Singapore to Sussex via France. *The Guardian*. https://www.theguardian.com/world/2020/feb/10/super-spreader-brought-coronavirus-from-singapore-to-sussex-via-france

Vicari, S., & Cappai, F. (2016). Health activism and the logic of connective action: A case study of rare disease patient organisations. *Information, Communication & Society*, *19*(11), 1653–1671.

Yang, G. (2020, February 3). *The digital radicals of Wuhan*. Center on Digital Culture and Society. https://u.osu.edu/mclc/2020/02/07/digital-radicals-of-wuhan/

Yang, G. (2021). Online lockdown diaries as endurance art. *Ai & Society*, 1–10.

Part 1

Theoretical Foundations

2 Digital Media, Participation and Citizenship

Introduction

This chapter draws on concepts and methods to investigate digital media, participation and citizenship. With "A story from the 1990s", the chapter starts by offering a view into early digital practices that questioned the role, essence and power structures surrounding "the media" and pre-digital forms of participation. It then steps further back in time to both map the origins of the digital media platforms where these practices emerged and reflect on the economic, social, and historical conditions affecting and shaping their development. This narration will be functional to understand shifts in 1) media structures, 2) content production, consumption, and usage and 3) participatory forms and potential. The second part of the chapter will focus on the everyday discursive practices enhanced by these shifts.

From Internet to Platforms: A Short History of Produsage (and Its Problems)

"Don't Hate the Media, Become the Media!"—A Story From the 1990s

It was November 1999 when a three-day protest in Seattle marked a turning point in the history of activism and a first milestone in that of *digital* activism, that is, of "political participation, activities and protests organised in digital networks beyond representational politics" (Karatzogianni, 2015, p. 1). A loose network of organisations and individuals from around the world launched the first of a number of street protests against international authorities, namely, the United Nations, the North Atlantic Treaty Organization and the European Union at the regional level; the World Trade Organization, the International Monetary Fund, the World Bank and the G8 at the global level (Tarrow, 2011; Vicari, 2014). While targeting international authorities, those activist networks advocated for economic, social, political and environmental justice and came to be known under the umbrella label of the Global Justice Movement (della Porta, 2006).

DOI: 10.4324/9780429469145-3

During the Seattle demonstrations against the World Trade Organization, the newly born Independent Media Centre, or Indymedia, launched the slogan "Don't hate the media, become the media"—one that would stick with activists worldwide for the following fifteen years. Indymedia was a rhizomatic network of both local groups and grass root news websites around the world advocating for bottom-up ways of news-making (Iannelli, 2016, p. 31). It strived to provide self-made coverage of protest events, with the 1999 "battle of Seattle" (Rojecki, 2011, pp. 88–89) working as a trial for all the transnational counter-summit protests that were to unfold over the following ten years or so. Like the Global Justice Movement itself, Indymedia kept developing at different levels of locality, with chapters opening around the world and working on the grass root coverage of social, economic and environmental issues at local, national and transnational levels. In 2011, Lievrouw was still writing of "175 Independent Media Centers (IMCs) worldwide" that aimed to create a "communication commons" (2011, p. 121).

Indymedia was at war with the legacy media; it aimed to become the antithesis to the vertical, top-down structure typical of traditional mainstream (mass) media systems as it produced and distributed crowdsourced, citizen-made news. It was participatory, activist and radical because it presented an alternative view in its being a "small-scale, low-budget, oppositional, and horizontal media" (Downing, 2003, p. 283). But what conditions led to the emergence of Indymedia?

From a sociotechnical point of view, Indymedia can be considered as one of the first and most radical global scale expressions of "produsage". To understand the meaning, unfolding and shortcomings of produsage as a conceptual tool to explore digital participatory practices, we need to take one further step back in time and trace the evolution of the digital media platforms we are familiar with today.

The Internet That Was

What we broadly refer to as "the Internet" has developed through different phases marked by economic, technical, and political factors. From being a small computer network used as a research tool by US tech elites in the 1970s, the Internet transitioned into being a "proto-commercial" (Curran & Seaton, 2010, p. 252) medium in the 1980s. Its infrastructure developed through the mushrooming of interconnected, grass root computer networks that hosted early discussion groups, namely usenets or virtual communities, driven by the American counterculture of the 1980s (Curran & Seaton, 2010, p. 260). Both usenets and virtual communities were developed to host discussions about a range of issues, with the former being geographically dispersed grassroot networks set up by students on university campuses and the latter working as local area networks bringing together social and political activists. This phase also saw the emergence of the first enthusiastic claims on the potential of the Internet, then mostly called "cyberspace", to enhance sociality and collaborative projects.

Ironically enough, though, some of the enthusiasm expressed then was already undermined by questions that sound extremely timely today. In 1993, Rheingold wrote of the virtual community (Whole Earth 'Lectronic Link'):

> Perhaps cyberspace is one of the informal public places where people can rebuild the aspects of community that were lost when the malt shop became a mall. Or perhaps cyberspace is precisely the wrong place to look for the rebirth of community, offering not a tool for conviviality but a life-denying simulacrum of real passion and true commitment to one another.
>
> (Rheingold, 2000 [1993], p. 10)

In fact, it was probably the parallel growth of commercial online services more than the spread of civically engaged grass root computer networks that brought significant, long-lasting changes. Following the release of the world wide web by the European research centre CERN, as "a free gift to the community" (Curran & Seaton, 2010, p. 263), commercial entities stepped in. Private investments in hardware and especially software development led to the introduction of user-friendly interfaces (e.g., Netscape, commercial graphical web browsers) that gradually turned the Internet from a niche research and *geek* tool into a medium accessible to unspecialised publics. As Curran & Seaton put it: "This transitional period closed with the sleeping giant of Microsoft awakening to the success of the web and assessing how best to profit from its growing popularity" (2010, p. 253).

The 1990s saw commercial content, especially net advertising, becoming gradually more prominent. While extending access, the new commercial regime saw the first consistent implementation of software licensing and the move online of traditional media corporations. The latter kept gaining power via increasingly gatekeeping usage and information flows through well-resourced websites, with search engines channelling users towards algorithmically defined prominent sources and gradually turning into all-inclusive portals (e.g., Yahoo). New forms of surveillance also emerged, though often unseen by users—for instance with the introduction of cookies and authentication processes—that enhanced both commercial and state surveillance.

Against this background, pre-market progressive countercultures and public service-style developments did not disappear, at times evolving in radical projects like Indymedia. However, commercially driven forces ultimately framed the Internet that would develop in the digital platforms we are mostly familiar with today.

From Media Consumers to Media Produsers

"Produsage" practices surfaced exactly in the mixed scenario of the 1990s, that is, with the "rise of the Internet as a *mass* medium-and as a mass medium which is significantly different from previous mass media" (Bruns, 2008, p. 13). The underlying argument here is that the traditional mass media system was structured around the producer, distributer, consumer linear model, where audiences, as consumers, have relatively little influence on content production and distribution. Of course, the cultural studies tradition has shown how audiences have always exerted a certain level of agency, especially in negotiating with or "decoding" (Hall, 1980) mass media content. As Iannelli sharply points out, cultural studies have long explored how minority publics challenge "hegemonic meanings" via their *own* interpretation of popular (mass) media content or how youth subcultures (e.g., punks, mods and hipsters) develop similar forms of resistance through the "*bricolage* of the ordinary" (Iannelli, 2016, p. 25, emphasis in original). However, the Internet seemed to escape the power imbalances underlying the technical and economic structures typical of traditional press and broadcast media systems: for the first time media content could be "pulled" by citizens, which also had unprecedented resources to produce and distribute their own content in collaborative, peer-to-peer projects (Bruns, 2008, p. 13). These dynamics also translated into new potential for information to be curated and further redistributed by citizens.

Overly enthusiastic views of produsage resonate with Negroponte's visionary picture in his 1995 "Being Digital", according to which: "Being digital will change the nature of mass media from a process of pushing bits at people to one of allowing people (or their computers) to pull at them" (p. 84). A picture that, bearing in mind the different commercialisation dynamics described above and the constant algorithmically informed "pushing" of promoted content in our contemporary social media feeds, sounds hyped and rather utopic. It is however undeniable that in the 1990s what was a mostly one-to-many, vertical (mass media) system of production and distribution started to work side by side with a much more nonlinear (online) system where consumers *could* turn into "produsers", that is, where consumers could access space and resources to produce, co-produce and distribute content.

Along with a number of scholars before and after him (e.g., Benkler, 2006; Castells, 2011), Bruns (2008) attributes this revolutionary shift in the traditional "mediasphere" to the networked structure of 1) the Internet as infrastructure, 2) the web as reticular content and 3) the groups of individuals gathering on the web as communities. Computer and content networks—children of the twentieth century "information technology revolution" (Castells, 2011)—did not suddenly *generate* a new form of sociality, that is, they did not generate a new way for people to relate to each other. However, they enhanced and accelerated an existing form of sociality that is not space-bound and is as likely to develop along weak ties (e.g., short lived, non-intimate relations) as it is along strong ones (e.g., family, long-lasting relations) (Rainie & Wellman, 2012, pp. 21–57). The new information and telecommunication technologies developing from the 1960s onwards enhanced this form of networked sociality by multiplying the opportunities to connect with others.

A key passage in the conceptualisation of produsage is that, while empowering this form of rhizomatic sociality, the twenty first century Internet normalised participatory models of content production where traditional role and power boundaries became increasingly fuzzy. As Bruns puts it: "Under a networked model . . . barriers to participation now are determined by questions of the individual's access to the network itself, and their capacity for understanding and adopting the prevailing protocols for effective contribution to 'hive mind' communities" (2008, p. 17). In conceptualising produsage, scholars were specifically interested in the new expressions of the "DIY culture of the web" (Curran & Seaton, 2010, p. 272) that surfaced in the twenty first century, that is, in the influence that 1980s and 1990s campus projects, grass root networks and countercultures had on the emergence of user-generated content (UGC) platforms, namely Web 2.0. Van Dijck frames this phase as one where online services shifted "from offering channels for networked communication to becoming interactive, two-way vehicles for networked sociality" (2013, p. 5). It is these platforms that, in a matter of less than a decade, evolved into the contemporary social media platforms.

Produsage Projects

While the Open Source movement drew upon the ideals and goals of the Internet's pre-market phase driven by the hacker community of the 1980s (Curran & Seaton, 2010, p. 387), citizen-journalism and knowledge sharing projects gradually emerged as new manifestations of Internet values and practices allowed by produsage dynamics. The label "citizen journalism" has come to address grass root, citizen-led instances of news-making and distribution like the Indymedia story presented at the beginning of the chapter. In reality, citizen journalism, while introducing "gatewatching" (Bruns, 2005) mechanisms whereby citizens select news of interest and share them with peers in networked communication flows, can take very different expressions. For instance, while Indymedia does represent a radical form of digital practice emerging within a transnational movement network, it would be hard to state the same for other examples of citizen journalism. Goode provides a rather compelling argument to downplay interpretations of citizen journalism that frame it as necessarily activist, let alone radical:

> Yahoo's purchase of Flickr . . . in 2005, Google's acquisition of Blogger.com in 2003 and YouTube in 2006, and MSNBC's acquisition of Newsvine in 2007 are salient examples. Even where there is clear institutional independence from "traditional" media, citizen journalism sites may draw (consciously or otherwise) on norms and traditions associated with mainstream journalism.
>
> (2009, p. 1289)

While blogs are a text and technological format typical of citizen journalism (Singer et al., 2011), wikis are at the centre of collaborative knowledge sharing, yet another expression of produsage. Wikipedia, launched in 2001 by the non-profit Wikimedia Foundation, presents itself as a "free online encyclopedia, created, edited, and verified by volunteers around the world, as well as many other vital community projects" (Wikimedia Foundation, 2020). Wikipedia is the key example of a long-lasting and ever-growing collaborative knowledge sharing project. Its content is produced, edited and updated by voluntary users, with content production being characterised by "the self-correcting mechanism of revision, a shared norm of adhering to factual accuracy, unobtrusive safe-guards and an academic tail of hypertextual links" (Curran & Seaton, 2010, p. 272). As such, Wikipedia follows the rules of "transparency, editability and community involvement" (Bruns, 2008, p. 138). Content on Wikipedia pages is published under free and open licenses. With Wikipedia's exponential growth, its contributors got gradually organised in a hierarchical order based on permission levels that would define what entries or edits to allow. In other words, Wikipedia's openness was made possible by the implementation of "a sophisticated technomanagerial system" assisted by "non-human content agents (or bots)" (Niederer & Van Dijck, 2010, p. 1369).

The examples of user-generated content discussed so far in relation to the open-source movement, citizen journalism practices, and collaborative knowledge sharing projects show that produsage does express itself via the production and sharing of information along horizontal and networked communication flows. However, framing produsage as necessarily alternative or radical would be misleading and would prevent us from comprehensively accounting for the different instances where users produce and share content on digital platforms. Yet again, this is primarily due to the mixed commercial and non-commercial forces that characterise contemporary digital media entities and practices. What, however, seems to cut across optimistic and critical views on the activist nature of produsage practices is the idea that, no matter the nature of the digital platforms hosting these practices and the organisations involved with them (e.g., commercial, governmental, and civic), they always imply participatory dynamics.

In updating his conceptualisation of produsage, Bruns hypothesises that digital community projects and commercial operators somehow reconciled with the emergence of twenty first century Western social media platforms (e.g., Facebook, Twitter):

> For example, engagement between journalism industry institutions and the citizen journalism communities, and alternative news discussion outside the industry, increasingly takes place not on the Websites of mainstream news sources . . . nor on the pages of citizen journalism sites and news blogs . . . but in the *neutral* spaces of Facebook and—especially—Twitter.
>
> (Bruns, 2012, p. 830, emphasis added)

But can contemporary social media platforms be considered neutral? To what extent are these platforms independent of economic and political forces? These questions require us to investigate participatory dynamics, user agency and platforms as closely interconnected.

Beyond Produsage: Participation, Agency and Platforms

A key question challenges views of produsage as inherently activist, that is, as necessarily challenging dominant social, cultural, and political dynamics (Lievrouw, 2011, p. 19): a question of agency. In other words, does relatively easy access to space and resources to produce and share content—namely, widened participatory potential—necessarily translate into user agency?

As signalled by the different expressions of produsage discussed in the previous section (e.g., Indymedia, citizen journalism hosted by commercial platforms, Wikipedia), "we need to account for the multifarious roles of users in a media environment where the boundaries between commerce, content and information are currently being redrawn" (Van Dijck, 2009, p. 42). In her 2009 work, Van Dijck draws attention to the different levels of engagement, or "active" participation, characterising UGC platforms, pointing to the very small percentage of users actually turning into produsers, that is, producing any content at all on these platforms. The question here is then on the extent to which *consuming* UGC content can be considered as an act of participation in itself or on whether similar "passive" forms of engagement turn platform users back into traditional content consumers. In other words, are these meaningless and disengaged expressions of "slacktivism" (Morozov, 2009) or "clicktivism" (Shulman, 2009) or are they rather legitimate and successful informal ways of political engagement (Christensen, 2011; Halupka, 2014; Karpf, 2010)? Can these forms of participation still take an activist turn? To address these questions, we also need to focus on the specific content being produced, shared, read and/or processed. The second part of the chapter will introduce a series of conceptual tools to investigate the discursive work navigating social media platforms and unpack the participatory nature of different practices (e.g., production, curation) related to it.

Perhaps most importantly, Van Dijck's (2009) analysis sheds light on the way UGC acquires value for users, platforms themselves and third parties. This work advocates for an interpretation of user agency that looks at the cultural, social, economic, technological, and legal aspects of UGC platforms as closely related. In so doing, it shifts the focus from users, or produsers, to platforms and their politics (Gillespie, 2010; Niederer & Van Dijck, 2010; Van Dijck, 2013; Van Dijck & Poell, 2013) preparing the grounds for "platform studies" research (e.g., Helmond, 2015; Plantin et al., 2018; Van Dijck et al., 2018).

Van Dijck (2013, p. 6) associates a key sociotechnical passage with the foundation of UGC platforms, one that sees Web 1.0's relatively heterogeneous communication channels turning into "applied services" that make the Internet more accessible but less tinkerable. Almost as if directly questioning Bruns' (2012) claims on social media neutrality, Van Dijck highlights that even if many big social media companies still want people to see them as mere communication channels, "this layer of applied platforms is anything but a neutral utility exploiting a generic resource (data)" (2013, p. 7).

Through social media, many everyday activities (e.g., gossiping, exchanging family pictures) have turned into permanent or semi-permanent digital traces, with this altering the nature of private and public communication. These very activities, and their digital traces, have then acquired increasing economic value: they are constantly translated into data that can be aggregated and analysed in different ways, not least to connect users with one another and with services and advertisements in *real time*. This process, labelled "datafication", enhances the circulation of information through platforms' application programming interfaces (APIs), which control access from third parties. In practice, datafication turns everyday activities into commodities, that is, into products that can be easily sold to and shared with third parties. Datafication also allows quantification, for instance of users' preferences or practices, that ultimately informs platforms' selection criteria, for example, of trending topics or influential users. According to Van Dijck et al. (2018), the tripartite process developing through datafication, commodification and selection ultimately defines contemporary (Western) societies as "platform societies".

But how does this process influence dynamics of participation? How do digital media practices aimed at challenging dominant social, cultural, and political views unfold in platform societies? A first and most evident impact is on visibility: *platformisation*, namely the tripartite process explained above, foregrounds certain content, while backgrounding others, on the basis of algorithmic choices. Only content that, for instance, makes it to Twitter's trending topic lists or Facebook personal news feeds is likely to reach wider social media publics and to be picked up by the mainstream media and ultimately intersect even wider publics. An example can help us understand these dynamics. In the late summer of 2011, the Occupy Wall Street protests were reaching high levels of participation, with Twitter being a key organisational and mobilisation channel (Tremayne, 2014). Yet, #occupywallstreet never made it to Twitter trending topic lists, not even in the cities where the protests were getting momentum (Gillespie, 2012; Van Dijck et al., 2018, p. 31). This was exclusively due to the way the Twitter Trend algorithm works in only selecting stories that register a *dramatic* increase in usage (Lotan, 2011; quoted in Van Dijck et al., 2018, p. 31). In August 2014, following the killing of Michael Brown by police officer Darren Wilson, the protests in the city of Ferguson became a Twitter trending topic for many users around the world while nothing similar was displayed by Facebook algorithmic news feeds (Tufekci, 2017, pp. 154–156). As a consequence, Twitter users would learn about police violence and protests in Ferguson while Facebook users would not. These stories suggest that only by taking into account platforms' mechanisms and their underlying politics, can we fully investigate the emergent, unfolding, nature and reach of contemporary participatory practices in the digital domain.

Data Activism and Digital Citizenship

While everyday digital media practices are increasingly shaped by the politics of platforms, the question stands of whether platform users may themselves try to resist or exploit these politics to foster social change, with the potential emergence of new activist dynamics. Milan and van der Velden (2016) discuss an epistemic shift in civil society, with data becoming a means to know the world and mobilise for change. The umbrella label of "data activism" indicates both proactive engagements with data, for instance in health activism (Milan & van der Velden, 2016), and resistance to normalised big data dynamics, like in forms of "digital citizenship" advocating for users' rights to privacy and personal data protection (Hintz et al., 2019, pp. 123–143). Drawing attention to contemporary understandings of how societies and societal structures work, Dencik (2018) frames data activism in terms of challenging how platform societies are organised and imagining new ways of living and experiencing life through data.

In reality, and in practice, data activism labels a number of participatory practices that have to do with data and datafication. Schrock (2016), for instance, frames contemporary "civic hacking" as a form of data activism deriving from the early twentieth century open-source movement, that itself links back to the hacker community of the 1980s. In particular, Schrock (2016) draws attention to the way hackers, as expert data users, can and do manipulate technology to foster social change and enhance democratic processes. While Schrock looks at experts, Kennedy (2018) shifts the focus to "non-expert citizens". Platformisation sets a hierarchy of power relations in the way data are produced, aggregated, used, and assigned economic value. Only an investigation of non-expert interpretations and feelings about datafication can then inform the implementation of just data practices. In other words: "How is datafication lived, felt and experienced by non-expert citizens before they start to develop the conditions or consider the possibility of activism in relation to data?" (Kennedy, 2018, p. 27).

In fact, data are part and parcel of our everyday life. In March 2020, digital diarist Guo Jing wrote of herself locked in Wuhan: "There was also a sense of anxiety from not knowing when it would end. I have looked at the *numbers* every day." (Kuo, 2020, emphasis mine). The numbers Jing refers to are the data that, from the end of February 2020, have become part of daily conversations and sometimes activist practices around the world: the numbers of Covid-19 testing, transmission rates, recovery and death, widely made available on digital platforms.

As we will see in the following sections, Kennedy's question is indeed extremely relevant to contemporary forms of activism—increasingly grounded in personal life stories and crowdsourced narratives of grievance and injustice (Bennett & Segerberg, 2013). The remainder of the chapter will shift the focus from media platforms to discursive dynamics: it will navigate theory and research focusing on *discursive* practices emerging in the digital media ecosystem.

Participation as Discursive Work: Public Sphere and Beyond

The question of if and how digital media can contribute to the emergence of a regenerated public sphere, in Habermasian terms, has now populated the sociological, media and communication terrains for over 20 years. As discussed in the previous section, the question is generally centred on the extent to which these platforms may enable (civic) agency, given the technological and socio-economic constraints that characterize both their development and context of origin (e.g., democratic countries, authoritarian regimes). The following sections will draw upon the rich and multidisciplinary scholarship that has specifically focused on online *discursive* actions differently challenging "dominant, expected, or accepted ways of doing society, culture, and politics" (Lievrouw, 2011, p. 19).

Due to platforms' API restrictions and the consequent constraints in data accessibility, most Western research developed in this direction has so far focused on Twitter. In fact, extensive debate has recently emerged on the deriving knock-on effect of the scholarly ability to provide comprehensive and reliable findings on the role of social media in contemporary societies (Rieder, 2016, 2018; Walker et al., 2019). Most of this work develops single-platform approaches to textual content, missing out on both the ecological dimension of the social media system and the contemporary turn to visual cultures (Leaver et al., 2020; Pearce et al., 2020; Serafinelli, 2018). Indeed, the empirical work discussed in the following sections draws upon this research strand and is affected by these very limitations. Where possible, attempts were made to incorporate studies focused on platforms other than Twitter, cross-platform research and visual analyses.

Internet and the Public Sphere

Early Internet studies explored ways to either apply Habermas' (1962) conceptualization of the public sphere to the online realm (see, for instance, Dahlberg, 2001; Emden, 2012, p. 66; Schneider, 1997), or use the public sphere as an ideal type, a metaphor against which to measure processes of democratisation (see, for instance, Papacharissi, 2008) and elaborate new theorizations for online informal political debate and civic agency (Dahlgren, 2000; Downey & Fenton, 2003; Fraser, 2007; Papacharissi, 2002). Studies from the second camp have interpreted the public sphere as an ideal realm of social life, where personal opinions on social and political issues can be shared, leading to public debate and, possibly, consensual deliberation. This research has often explored the renegotiation of private and public domains, in particular when individuals challenge the public agenda determined by legacy news producers.

In framing the concept of "civic culture", Dahlgren (2005, pp. 148–150), for instance, advances a threefold interpretation of the public sphere concept, organised along structural, representational, and interactional dimensions. The structural dimension involves the social, economic, and political availability of infrastructures that channel flows of information. The representational dimension refers to if, how and to what extent different publics get represented in public debates. The interactional dimension concerns reciprocity, namely, the emergence of the dialogical debate characteristic of healthy public sphere dynamics. As I previously discussed in the context of research exploring the early Cuban blogosphere (Vicari, 2015), representational and interactional dimensions are mostly dependent on the structural one, namely: for publics to be represented and develop internal and outfacing dialogue, structural availability is a sine qua non condition.

In his investigation of the Internet context prior to the advent of social media platforms, Benkler (2006) centres his theorisation of the "networked public sphere" on what Dahlgren (2005) defines as the "structural dimension" of the public sphere, namely, Internet networks. In line with Bruns (2008), Benkler's aim is that of measuring the extent to which networked flows of information and communication could enable more civic agency than the linear flows typical of mainstream media systems. Ultimately, Benkler's position asserts a positive relationship between Internet usage and potential for civic action but has had to face a line of strong criticisms. In fact, parallel research has drawn attention to a number of issues that are still relevant today, namely, the uneven levels of Internet access across social groups and cultural contexts, the lack of reciprocity in most online communication (Bohman, 2004, p. 135; Papacharissi, 2008, pp. 234–235), the online information overload that leads to the fragmentation of online publics (Habermas, 2006, pp. 423–424 n. 3; Sustein, 2009), the polarisation of discourse practices (Benkler, 2006, p. 235), the commercialisation of online channels of information and communication (Noam, 2005; Papacharissi, 2008, pp. 235–236) and dynamics of centralisation, or how only few websites receive most readers' attention (Benkler, 2006, pp. 235–236; Hindman, 2009). The arguments used to counter these criticisms primarily draw upon the ever-increasing Internet penetration rates, not least via mobile devices, and again on network behaviour dynamics, or the "filtering, accreditation, and synthesis mechanisms" (Benkler, 2006, p. 271) allowed by networked topologies. Benkler (2006) pushes his argument even further by saying that "because of these emerging systems, the networked information economy is solving the information overload and discourse fragmentation concerns without introducing the distortion of the mass-media model" (p. 271).

While the digital ecosystem explored with these early theorisations has now dramatically changed, in the course of the next sections we will see that they are still at the core of much of the current debate on public sphere and counterpublic dynamics investigated in the context of contemporary social media platforms.

Social Media, Issue Publics and Crowdsourced Discourse

Past the first wave of Internet studies, which primarily focused on Web 1.0 and early instances of Web 2.0 (e.g., blogs and blogospheres), the coming to prominence of contemporary digital platforms awakened interest in "performative" publics[1] (Abercrombie & Longhurst, 1998). In specific terms, with social media platforms becoming ubiquitous in everyday life, the concept of "issue public" has become central to research interested in the discursive work developed by social media users around issues of public relevance. The concept—originally introduced by political scientist Philip Converse in the 1960s—is generally used to address groupings of platform users producing and sharing content related to a specific issue.

After Tremayne and colleagues' (2006) work on political blogospheres, research on issue publics has primarily focused on Twitter conversations about major events and breaking news. To provide a theoretical underpinning for this work, Bruns and Highfield (2015) stress that Twitter issue publics form in relation to "short-term aspects" that motivate public debate on a specific topic. Bruns and Burgess even introduce the concept of "ad-hoc publics" to describe Twitter "discursive communities around a central shared interest", highlighting that "What particularly allows Twitter and its hashtag communities to stand out from . . . other spaces for issue publics is its ability to respond with great speed to emerging issues and acute events" (2011, p. 11).

Social media research has explored very different types of issue publics emerging on Twitter: Yardi and Boyd's (2010) work, for instance, analyses the issue public developing in response to the shooting of late-term abortion doctor Tiller in the US, while Pearce and colleagues (2014) investigate the issue public commenting the publication of the 2013 IPCC Working Group 1 Report, "a critical event in the societal debate about climate change". As I will further discuss in Chapter 6, in my own work on health-related issue publics (Vicari, 2017), I shift the focus on long-lived issue publics forming around specific health conditions. Similarly, Sandover et al. (2018) explore the long-lasting Twitter debate focused on the state-sanctioned cull of wild badgers in England. But what is the nature of the discursive work produced within social media issue publics?

As in early Web 2.0 studies, social media research has drawn attention to the way platforms enhance the organisation of shared knowledge, with individuals and collective actors participating in the development of collaborative information and mobilisatiom dynamics. Exploring contemporary instances of activism, Bennett and Segerberg (2013) distinguish between two new forms of digitally-driven civic engagement: "organizationally enabled" and "crowd-enabled" "connective action." In organizationally enabled connective action, social media platforms, or "digitally networking mechanisms", allow organizations to mobilise individuals around issues of public relevance. In crowd-enabled connective action, people use digitally networking mechanisms to join activist campaigns without the intermediation of traditional organizations. The logic of connective action draws upon the idea that digital media in general, and social media platforms in particular, allow the emergence of collaborative processes based on shared understandings of grievance. These shared understandings, according to Bennett and Segerberg (2013), are grounded on personal stories, namely "personal action frames". In other words, in crowd-sourced connective action, people do not necessarily engage in campaigns or activist debates on social media and elsewhere because of their political party affiliation or as members of a pressure group (e.g., Greenpeace); they do so because the campaign or debate resonates to their life story. Bennett and Segerberg (2013, p. 7) use "We are the 99%", the slogan launched in 2011 by the Occupy protests in the United States, to make their point. The slogan became the title of a blog on microblogging service Tumblr, attracting hundreds of posts by people who wrote their personal story that made them part of the 99%.

Ultimately, Bennett and Segerberg's (2013) research questions the continuing significance of "collective identities" (Melucci, 1995) in contemporary activism, asserting a decline in the importance of the shared belief systems typical of traditional social movements, protest and activism. This view has faced a rather strong backlash among social movement scholars, with a line of key authors advocating for the continuing significance of collective actors and identities (Bakardjieva, 2015; Gerbaudo & Treré, 2015; Kavada, 2015; Milan, 2015). However, whether we define contemporary digital activism in terms of new expressions of activist collective actors (Bakardjieva, 2015; Gerbaudo & Treré, 2015; Kavada, 2015; Milan, 2015) or personalised forms of civic engagement that lead to shared action (Bennett & Segerberg, 2013), we are faced with the challenge to understand power relations among the entities involved (e.g., individuals, organisations) and meaning making in networked communication flows.

In the attempt to describe the nature of social media content production that may as well happen in activist contexts, Hermida (2010) defines Twitter's functionality as that of a "collective intelligence" and an "awareness system" (p. 298)—that is, one that allows users to incorporate information and knowledge deriving from varied sources, challenging traditional protocols of public communication. The idea of a Twitter-generated "awareness system" obviously backgrounds questions of information reliability while foregrounding issues of knowledge inclusivity. In fact, it has been shown that Twitter does not necessarily enhance intentionally collaborative processes (Kwak et al., 2010; Vicari, 2013), but does show potential for broadcasting and gatekeeping of user-generated or user-selected content (Bastos et al., 2013; Benkler, 2006, p. 271; Boyd et al., 2010; Bruns & Burgess, 2012; Jackson & Foucault Welles, 2015, 2016; Meraz & Papacharissi, 2013; Tremayne, 2014). This happens via mechanisms that are platform-bound, that is, mechanisms that express themselves via the use of conversational (i.e., @, RT) and tagging (i.e., #) markers.

Crowdsourced dynamics happen within a "hybrid media system" (Chadwick, 2017), one where "a global integration of different types and systems of media—personal and mass, national and international" (Bennett et al., 2014, p. 232) sees content bouncing back and forth between legacy media and social media platforms. For instance, Papacharissi and de Fatima Oliveira (2012) have defined Twitter's functionality as that of a "news reporting mechanism"—or one that allows the integration of different forms of news reporting. The "ambient" aspect of Twitter (Bruns & Burgess, 2012; Hermida, 2010) reveals itself exactly in this overlapping of different levels of communication and media practices: from background, always on, "mundane and phatic" posting, to sudden shifts in vocabulary, topic, tone, and targets when important news enters the Twittersphere (Bruns & Burgess, 2012, p. 802). Not only does this happen in second screen (Giglietto & Selva, 2014; Iannelli & Giglietto, 2014) or dual screening (Vaccari et al., 2015) practices—where social media users live-comment mainstream media content. Research has shown that this also occurs, for instance, in microblogging about events of public interest (Bennett et al., 2014; Jackson & Foucault Welles, 2015; Papacharissi & de Fatima Oliveira, 2012; Vicari, 2013).

In sum, to investigate the shape of social media discursive work, empirical studies have drawn attention to two dimensions that enhance both crowdsourcing and hybrid dynamics: the curation of content produced and shared in social media streams and the way meaning is constructed within these streams. Research interested in the latter is now also starting to explore the rise of visual cultures—and countercultures.

Curating Content on Social Media: The Rise of New Counterpublics?

Marres and Gerlitz (2016) advocate for social media issue mappings that use "empiricist" and "affirmative" approaches, that is, that consider the use of digital mechanisms (e.g., platform-bound communication practices) as a constitutive element of knowledge production in issue publics. Twitter discursive work, for instance, expresses itself in the constant live-streaming of 280-character posts where conversational markers can facilitate networking dynamics among users. Retweeting implies exposing someone's message to a wider public and @ is a conversational marker that allows users to mention or direct posts to other users, sustaining "a high level of interactivity and engagement" (Meraz & Papacharissi, 2013, p. 140). In the ecology of live-streaming, these mechanisms entail drawing attention to a set of privileged Twitter users, more specifically, to their username (in the case of RT and @) and/or to content tweeted by them (in the case of RT). Those who engage in RT or @ use have been defined as "broadcasters" because they amplify other users' voice and/or identity. Bennett, Segerberg and Walker frame these mechanisms as part of the broader process of "curation", which entails "the preservation, maintenance, and sorting of digital assets" (2014, p. 239).

Drawing upon work by Smith et al. (2014), Jackson and Foucault Welles (2015, 2016) add to the understanding of Twitter broadcasting by describing #myNYPD and #Ferguson Twitter streams as "broadcast networks". Both networks emerged on Twitter and spread to other social media platforms in response to police brutality in the US. The former hijacked a public relations campaign by the New York City Police Department in April 2014 while the latter developed in response to the killing of Michael Brown in the city of Ferguson in August 2014. Broadcast networks, write Jackson and Foucault Welles, have "a distinctive hub-and-spoke structure where most nodes in the network radiate out from a small number of central nodes" (2015, p. 938). According to the authors, Twitter broadcast networks generate conversational space for minority viewpoints that would otherwise be missed in mainstream public sphere dynamics. Jackson and Foucault Welles go as far as to define Twitter broadcast networks as "networked counterpublics", that is, the ultimate, networked expression of Fraser's (1990) "parallel discursive arenas where members of subordinated social groups invent and circulate counterdiscourses, which in turn permit them to formulate oppositional interpretations of their identities, interests, and needs" (p. 67).

In an issue-based Twitter stream, while broadcasters extend the lifespan of successful Twitter content, gatekeepers are Twitter users brought to prominence via the use of conversational markers. In other words, users whose messages are most frequently retweeted or shared or whose handle is most frequently mentioned via the @ marker become the gatekeepers—or *influencers*—of an issue public. As Bastos and colleagues (2013, p. 3) suggest, "Gatekeeping is still a key mechanism in digital networks, only now it has been redesigned to incorporate a multitude of senders and receivers". In fact, by highlighting the networked nature of discursive dynamics on social media platforms, the concept of "networked gatekeeping" (Meraz & Papacharissi, 2013) underlines the potential turning of traditionally non-elite actors into primary sources of information.

Most of the research presented here and in the previous section primarily explores the materiality of digital media platforms and its impact on users' potential to connect with one another and bolster social change. The transient nature of this potential suggests that digital media platforms shape the construction of "contentious publicness" (Kavada & Poell, 2021), namely, they influence both how individuals participate in public conversations and what public conversations they participate in.

Affective Dynamics and Hashtag Activism

It is expressions of sentiment that often mobilise, connect, or disconnect publics on social media. Papacharissi (2015) introduces the concept of "affective publics" to point to the relevance of individual and collective emotions in social media issue publics. The expressions of sentiment emerging on these platforms develop through the blending of opinions, facts, and feelings in always-on or intermittent discursive streams. As a matter of fact, mainstream social media platforms are designed to nurture, datafy and quantify public emotion—as environments where users' sentiment can be managed and algorithmically manipulated (Wahl-Jorgensen, 2019, p. 165).

In the emotionally driven assemblages happening within social media discursive streams, hashtags play the central role of enhancing, defining and associating narratives around specific issues or events. In blending emotion-tuned content, hashtags ultimately help the formation of issue publics: "In scenarios where communities converge on a selected hashtag to represent an issue or topic, such hashtags aid in the creation of an ad hoc issue public, collating tweets along a specific, topical dimension" (Meraz & Papacharissi, 2013, p. 143). Clearly, issue publics are in primis "discourse communities" as they emerge in a context where language plays a leading role in shaping sociality (Zappavigna, 2011).

Research has explored hashtags as "framing devices" (Gamson & Modigliani, 1989), namely as rhetorical tools used to form and communicate interpretations and narratives of issues and events. It was Bateson (1972) who first conceptualised frames as ways to understand messages, namely, processes or "schemata of interpretation" (Goffman, 1974) by which we select and retain parts of a message to shape and understand the message itself. Hashtags, as framing devices, help platform users to understand, organise and amplify—or dismiss—messages. Meraz and Papacharissi (2013) apply frame theory to the analysis of Twitter hashtags using frame concepts to explore, map, and interpret prominent narratives during the 2011 Egypt uprisings. Their day-by-day investigation shows that quantitatively prominent hashtags—and hence dominant narratives—converged around the most significant events occurring during the protests. Users converged on a common interpretation of the events by using factual information like key dates, geographic locations, and public figures (Meraz & Papacharissi, 2013, p. 153). Dahlberg-Grundberg and Lindgren (2014) look at the use of tweets with multiple hashtags as an indication of "frame articulation" and "frame alignment", that is, the association of previously disconnected issues. In their work on the Idlenomore movement in Canada, they suggest that the use of #idlenomore with other activist hashtags (e.g., #ows for Occupy Wall Street and #Egypt for the 2011 Egypt uprising) shows a sort of symbolic association between instances of activism, which enhances the emergence of social movement narratives spanning across cultures and places.

Given their semantic (Meraz & Papacharissi, 2013) and communitarian (Zappavigna, 2011; Rambukkana, 2015) potential, hashtags have come to label a new form of digital activist practice, that of "hashtag activism". Hashtag activism describes issue publics that challenge dominant political, social, or cultural views, and are united through a hashtagged word, phrase, or sentence (e.g., #BlackLivesMatter) (Jackson et al., 2020; Yang, 2016b). In line with the frame analyses presented above, Yang's work stresses hashtags' symbolic power, but also draws specific attention to their "rhetorical agency"—the ability to convey and contain counter messages that have high cultural relevance, especially to minority groups. While aiming at advancing specific narratives, however, hashtag activism is also subject to hashtags' "protean" nature, namely it can be easily hijacked or manipulated by third parties that manage to produce noise in activist hashtagged streams, blurring their intended message.

Visual Cultures and Countercultures

The mediation of issues or events that happens within issue publics develops via the assemblage of words, images, audio, video, and other affective devices that we use to understand the world and turn it into "pictures in our heads" (Papacharissi, 2015, p. 130). In fact, the affective dimension of social media discursive sociality (Papacharissi, 2015) and platform architectures (Wahl-Jorgensen, 2019) thrives with the use of visual content.

Digital scholarship interested in "participatory cultures" (Cammaerts, 2007; Jenkins, 2006) has shown that social media platforms allow the unprecedented circulation and visibility of user-manipulated visuals with activist purposes. These visual artefacts are often used to dispute the cultural models that emerge in dominant languages and cultural codes (e.g., in relation to genre, race, religion, and lifestyles). Jenkins (2006) has long stressed on citizens' skills to manipulate media content with the aim of foregrounding critical and/or marginalised opinions. Jenkins' work likens the "photoshop for democracy" emerging in the early Web 2.0 domain to the grassroots resistance described by Dery's (1993) "culture jamming", namely, the "'DIY media' and their strategies for gathering consensus through the manipulation of signs such as media hacking, terror art, and semiological guerrilla tactics" (Iannelli, 2016, p. 58).

The digital jamming of visual content has been investigated as an activist practice that enhances the circulation of critical views *across* media platforms (Deuze, 2010; Gray, 2012), a phenomenon called "spreadability" (Jenkins et al., 2013). These dynamics have been specifically explored in relation to contemporary memes—"(post)modern folklore, in which shared norms and values are constructed through cultural artifacts such as Photoshopped images or urban legends that is, multimodal artefacts that mix visual and textual elements" (Shifman, 2014, p. 15). Milner's (2013) work, for instance, shows that Occupy Wall Street memes enhanced "pop polivocality", namely, they attracted commentaries and debates from multiple perspectives, often generating complex public conversations on Reddit, Tumblr, and 4chan. Similar forms of memetic countervisuality have also been explored in single-platform studies. Frazer and Carlson (2017), for instance, discuss how Australian Aboriginal activists produce and broadcast anti-colonial messages on Facebook. Jensen et al. (2020) show how memes enhanced the overlaying of popular culture, resistance, and solidarity on Twitter during the 2015 Brussels lockdown due to anti-terrorism measures.

In their discussion of visual social media cultures, Leaver et al. (2020, pp. 151–152) explore initiatives that directly engage with platforms' norms to raise social awareness. In their analysis of Instagram as a "conduit for communication", they describe the @barbiesaviour account as a visual means to criticise white saviour narratives via satirical travelogues. An even more platform-bound form of civic agency is represented by the use of Instagram filters designed to counter social inequalities in Singapore, where the #YellowHelmetChallenge filter allows the superimposition of a yellow-coloured helmet—a symbol of foreign underpaid workers—on a selfie.

Hence, contemporary social media platforms offer potential for old and new visual expressions, often influenced or shaped by platform norms. These norms have been shown to both enhance creative expressions and satirical potential (Leaver et al., 2020) and reproduce hierarchical structures of power grounded in the datafication and selection dynamics presented earlier (Neumayer &

Rossi, 2018). This points to the increasing relevance of visual content in both social media communication practices and participatory cultures.

Conclusion

This chapter has reviewed key concepts to investigate digital media, participation, and citizenship. The development of contemporary digital media platforms has been shaped by economic, social and historical conditions affecting media structures, modes of production, consumption, usage and, ultimately, forms of participation. In turn, these developments have paved the way for old and new discursive potential for public sphere and counterpublic dynamics. Most importantly, this chapter shows that contemporary participatory practices are increasingly shaped by platforms and their politics. In the next chapter, we will move on to address theories and debates directly focusing on participatory practices emerging in the context of health advocacy and activism.

Note

1. For a relevant discussion, see Iannelli (2016, pp. 21–28).

Reference List

Abercrombie, N., & Longhurst, B. J. (1998). *Audiences: A sociological theory of performance and imagination*. SAGE Publications Ltd.

Bakardjieva, M. (2015). Do clouds have politics? Collective actors in social media land. *Information, Communication & Society*, *18*(8), 983–990.

Bastos, M. T., Raimundo, R. L. G., & Travitzki, R. (2013). Gatekeeping Twitter: Message diffusion in political hashtags. *Media, Culture & Society*, *35*(2), 260–270.

Bateson, G. (1972). *Steps to an ecology of mind: Collected essays in anthropology, psychiatry, evolution, and epistemology*. University of Chicago Press.

Benkler, Y. (2006). *The wealth of networks: How social production transforms markets and freedom*. Yale University Press.

Bennett, W. L., & Segerberg, A. (2013). *The logic of connective action: Digital media and the personalization of contentious politics*. Cambridge University Press.

Bennett, W. L., Segerberg, A., & Walker, S. (2014). Organization in the crowd: Peer production in large-scale networked protests. *Information, Communication & Society*, *17*(2), 232–260.

Bohman, J. (2004). Expanding dialogue: The Internet, the public sphere and prospects for transnational democracy. *The Sociological Review*, *52*(1_suppl), 131–155.

Boyd, D., Golder, S., & Lotan, G. (2010, January). Tweet, tweet, retweet: Conversational aspects of retweeting on twitter. In *2010 43rd Hawaii International Conference on System Sciences* (pp. 1–10). IEEE.

Bruns, A. (2005). *Gatewatching: Collaborative online news production* (Vol. 26). Peter Lang.

Bruns, A. (2008). *Blogs, Wikipedia, Second Life, and beyond: From production to produsage* (Vol. 45). Peter Lang.

Bruns, A. (2012). Reconciling community and commerce? Collaboration between produsage communities and commercial operators. *Information, Communication & Society*, *15*(6), 815–835.

Bruns, A., & Burgess, J. E. (2011, August). The use of Twitter hashtags in the formation of ad hoc publics. In *Proceedings of the 6th European Consortium for Political Research (ECPR) General Conference 2011*.

Bruns, A., & Burgess, J. (2012). Researching news discussion on Twitter: New methodologies. *Journalism Studies*, *13*(5–6), 801–814.

Bruns, A., & Highfield, T. (2015). Is Habermas on Twitter? Social media and the public sphere. In *The Routledge companion to social media and politics* (pp. 56–73). Routledge.

Cammaerts, B. (2007). Jamming the political: Beyond counter-hegemonic practices. *Continuum*, *21*(1), 71–90.

Castells, M. (2011). *The rise of the network society* (Vol. 12). John Wiley & Sons.

Chadwick, A. (2017). *The hybrid media system: Politics and power*. Oxford University Press.

Christensen, H. S. (2011). Political activities on the Internet: Slacktivism or political participation by other means? *First Monday*, *16*(2), fm.v16i2.3336.

Curran, J., & Seaton, J. (2010). *Power without responsibility* (7th ed.). Routledge.

Dahlberg, L. (2001). Computer-mediated communication and the public sphere: A critical analysis. *Journal of Computer-Mediated Communication*, *7*(1), JCMC714.

Dahlgren, P. (2000). The Internet and the democratization of civic culture. *Political Communication*, *17*(4), 335–340.

Dahlgren, P. (2005). The Internet, public spheres, and political communication: Dispersion and deliberation. *Political Communication*, *22*(2), 147–162.

Dahlberg-Grundberg, M., & Lindgren, S. (2014). Translocal frame extensions in a networked protest: Situating the #IdleNoMore hashtag. *IC: Revista Científica de Información y Comunicación*, *11*, 49–77.

della Porta, D. (2006). *Globalization from below: Transnational activists and protest networks*. University of Minnesota Press.

Dencik, L. (2018). Surveillance realism and the politics of imagination: Is there no alternative? *Krisis: Journal for Contemporary Philosophy*, *2018*(1), 31–43.

Dery, M. (1993). *Culture jamming: Hacking, slashing, and sniping in the empire of signs* (Vol. 25). Open Media.

Deuze, M. (2010). Survival of the mediated. *Journal of Cultural Science*, *3*, 1–11.

Downey, J., & Fenton, N. (2003). New media, counter publicity and the public sphere. *New Media & Society*, *5*(2), 185–202.

Downing, J. (2003). Radical media and globalization. In *The globalization of corporate media hegemony* (pp. 283–293). State University of New York Press.

Emden, C. J. (2012). Epistemic publics. On the trading zone of knowledge. In Emden, C. J. & Midgley, D. (Eds.) *Beyond Habermas: Democracy, knowledge and the public sphere* (pp. 63–86). Berghahn Books.

Fraser, N. (1990). Rethinking the public sphere: A contribution to the critique of actually existing democracy. *Social Text*, *25/26*, 56–80.

Fraser, N. (2007). Transnational public sphere: Transnationalizing the public sphere: On the legitimacy and efficacy of public opinion in a post-Westphalian world. *Theory, Culture & Society*, *24*(4), 7–30.

Frazer, R., & Carlson, B. (2017). Indigenous memes and the invention of a people. *Social Media + Society*, *3*(4), 2056305117738993.

Gamson, W. A., & Modigliani, A. (1989). Media discourse and public opinion on nuclear power: A constructionist approach. *American Journal of Sociology*, *95*(1), 1–37.

Gerbaudo, P., & Treré, E. (2015). In search of the “we” of social media activism: Introduction to the special issue on social media and protest identities. *Information, Communication & Society*, *18*(8), 865–871.

Giglietto, F., & Selva, D. (2014). Second screen and participation: A content analysis on a full season dataset of tweets. *Journal of Communication, 64*, 260–277.

Gillespie, T. (2010). The politics of "platforms". *New Media & Society, 12*(3), 347–364.

Gillespie, T. (2012). Can an algorithm be wrong? *Limn, 1*(2).

Goffman, E. (1974). *Frame analysis*. Harper Colophon.

Goode, L. (2009). Social news, citizen journalism and democracy. *New Media & Society, 11*(8), 1287–1305.

Gray, J. (2012). Of snowspeeders and Imperial Walkers: Fannish play at the Wisconsin protests. *Transformative Works and Cultures, 10*, 1–7.

Habermas, J. (1989 [1962]). *The structural transformation of the public sphere: An inquiry into a category of a bourgeois society*. The MIT Press.

Habermas, J. (2006). Political communication in media society: Does democracy still enjoy an epistemic dimension? The impact of normative theory on empirical research. *Communication Theory, 16*, 411–426.

Hall, S. (1980). Encoding/decoding in television discourse. In Hall, S., Hobson, D., Lowe, A., & Willis, P. (Eds.) *Culture, Media, Language* (pp. 128–138). Hutchinson.

Halupka, M. (2014). Clicktivism: A systematic heuristic. *Policy & Internet, 6*(2), 115–132.

Helmond, A. (2015). The platformization of the web: Making web data platform ready. *Social Media + Society, 1*(2), 2056305115603080.

Hermida, A. (2010). Twittering the news: The emergence of ambient journalism. *Journalism Practice, 4*(3), 297–308.

Hindman, M. (2009). *The myth of digital democracy*. Princeton University Press.

Hintz, A., Dencik, L., & Wahl-Jorgensen, K. (2019). *Digital citizenship in a datafied society*. John Wiley & Sons.

Iannelli, L. (2016). *Hybrid politics: Media and participation*. Sage.

Iannelli, L., & Giglietto, F. (2014). Hybrid spaces of politics: The 2013 general elections in Italy, between talk shows and Twitter. *Information, Communication & Society, 18*, 1006–1021.

Jackson, S., Bailey, M., & Welles, B. (2020). *#hashtagactivism: Networks of race and gender justice*. MIT Press.

Jackson, S., & Foucault Welles, B. (2015). Hijacking #myNYPD: Social media dissent and networked counterpublics. *Journal of Communication, 65*, 932–952.

Jackson, S., & Foucault Welles, B. (2016). #Ferguson is everywhere: Initiators in emerging counterpublic networks. *Information, Communication & Society, 19*, 397–418.

Jenkins, H. (2006). *Fans, bloggers, and gamers: Exploring participatory culture*. New York University Press.

Jenkins, H., Ford, S., & Green, J. (2013). *Spreadable media: Creating value and meaning in a networked culture*. New York University Press.

Jensen, M. S., Neumayer, C., & Rossi, L. (2020). "Brussels will land on its feet like a cat": Motivations for memefying# Brusselslockdown. *Information, Communication & Society, 23*(1), 59–75.

Karatzogianni, A. (2015). *Firebrand waves of digital activism 1994–2014: The rise and spread of hacktivism and cyberconflict*. Springer.

Karpf, D. (2010). Online political mobilization from the advocacy group's perspective: Looking beyond clicktivism. *Policy & Internet, 2*(4), 7–41.

Kavada, A. (2015). Creating the collective: Social media, the Occupy Movement and its constitution as a collective actor. *Information, Communication & Society, 18*(8), 872–886.

Kavada, A., & Poell, T. (2021). From counterpublics to contentious publicness: Tracing the temporal, spatial, and material articulations of popular protest through social media. *Communication Theory*, *31*(2), 190–208.

Kennedy, H., (2018). Living with data: Aligning data studies and data activism through a focus on everyday experiences of datafication. *Krisis: Journal for Contemporary Philosophy*, (1).

Kuo, L. (2020, March 15). Write a diary, take action: Hubei residents on fighting coronavirus anxiety. *The Guardian*. www.theguardian.com/world/2020/mar/15/write-a-diary-take-action-hubei-residents-on-fighting-coronavirus-anxiety

Kwak, H., Lee, C., Park, H., & Moon, S. (2010, April). What is Twitter, a social network or a news media? In *Proceedings of the 19th International Conference on World Wide Web* (pp. 591–600).

Leaver, T., Highfield, T., & Abidin, C. (2020). *Instagram: Visual social media cultures*. John Wiley & Sons.

Lievrouw, L. (2011). *Alternative and activist new media*. Polity.

Lotan, G. (2011). Data reveals that "occupying" Twitter Trending Topics is harder than it looks! *Giladlotan.com, 12*.

Marres, N., & Gerlitz, C. (2016). Interface methods: Renegotiating relations between digital social research, STS and sociology. *The Sociological Review*, *64*(1), 21–46.

Melucci, A. (1995). The process of collective identity. *Social Movements and Culture*, *4*, 41–63.

Meraz, S., & Papacharissi, Z. (2013). Networked gatekeeping and networked framing on #Egypt. *The International Journal of Press/Politics*, *18*, 138–166.

Milan, S. (2015). From social movements to cloud protesting: The evolution of collective identity. *Information, Communication & Society*, *18*(8), 887–900.

Milan, S., & Van der Velden, L. (2016). The alternative epistemologies of data activism. *Digital Culture & Society*, *2*(2), 57–74.

Milner, R. M. (2013). Pop polyvocality: Internet memes, public participation, and the Occupy Wall Street Movement. *International Journal of Communication*, *7*, 34.

Morozov, E. (2009). The brave new world of slacktivism. *Foreign Policy*, *19*(5).

Negroponte, N. (1995). *Being digital*. Hodder & Stoughton.

Neumayer, C., & Rossi, L. (2018). Images of protest in social media: Struggle over visibility and visual narratives. *New Media & Society*, *20*(11), 4293–4310.

Niederer, S., & Van Dijck, J. (2010). Wisdom of the crowd or technicity of content? Wikipedia as a sociotechnical system. *New Media & Society*, *12*(8), 1368–1387.

Noam, E. M. (2005). Why the Internet is bad for democracy. *Communications of the ACM*, *48*(10), 57–58.

Papacharissi, Z. (2002). The virtual sphere: The Internet as a public sphere. *New Media & Society*, *4*(1), 9–27.

Papacharissi, Z. (2008). The virtual sphere 2.0: The Internet, the public sphere, and beyond. In *Routledge handbook of Internet politics* (pp. 246–261). Routledge.

Papacharissi, Z. (2015). *Affective publics: Sentiment, technology, and politics*. Oxford University Press.

Papacharissi, Z., & de Fatima Oliveira, M. (2012). Affective news and networked publics: The rhythms of news storytelling on #Egypt. *Journal of Communication*, *62*, 266–282.

Pearce, W., Holmberg, K., Hellsten, I., Nerlich, B., & Amblard, F. (2014). Climate change on Twitter: Topics, communities and conversations about the 2013 IPCC Working Group 1 Report. *PLoS One*, *9*(4), e94785.

Pearce, W., Özkula, S. M., Greene, A. K., Teeling, L., Bansard, J. S., Omena, J. J., & Rabello, E. T. (2020). Visual cross-platform analysis: Digital methods to research social media images. *Information, Communication & Society*, *23*(2), 161–180.

Plantin, J. C., Lagoze, C., Edwards, P. N., & Sandvig, C. (2018). Infrastructure studies meet platform studies in the age of Google and Facebook. *New Media & Society*, *20*(1), 293–310.

Rainie, H., & Wellman, B. (2012). *Networked: The new social operating system* (Vol. 419). MIT Press.

Rambukkana, N. (2015). *Hashtag publics: The power and politics of discursive networks*. Peter Lang Publishing.

Rheingold, H. (2000 [1993]). *The virtual community: Homesteading on the electronic frontier*. MIT Press.

Rieder, B. (2016). Closing APIs and the public scrutiny of very large online platforms. *Politics of Systems Blog*, *27*. http://thepoliticsofsystems.net/2016/05/closing-apis-and-the-public-scrutiny-of-very-large-online-platforms/

Rieder, B. (2018). Facebook's app review and how independent research just got a lot harder. *The Politics of Systems Blog*. http://thepoliticsofsystems.net/2018/08/facebooks-app-review-and-how-independent-research-just-got-a-lot-harder/

Rojecki, A. (2011). Leaderless crowds, self-organizing publics, and virtual masses: The new media politics of dissent. In *Transnational protests and the media* (pp. 87–97). Peter Lang.

Sandover, R., Kinsley, S., & Hinchliffe, S. (2018). A very public cull: The anatomy of an online issue public. *Geoforum*, *97*, 106–118.

Schneider, S. M. (1997). *Expanding the public sphere through computer-mediated communication: Political discussion about abortion*. Massachusetts Institute of Technology.

Schrock, A. R. (2016). Civic hacking as data activism and advocacy: A history from publicity to open government data. *New Media & Society*, *18*(4), 581–599.

Serafinelli, E. (2018). *Digital life on Instagram: New social communication of photography*. Emerald Group Publishing.

Shifman, L. (2014). The cultural logic of photo-based meme genres. *Journal of Visual Culture*, *13*, 340–358.

Shulman, S. W. (2009). The case against mass e-mails: Perverse incentives and low quality public participation in US federal rulemaking. *Policy & Internet*, *1*(1), 23–53.

Singer, J. B., Domingo, D., Heinonen, A., Hermida, A., Paulussen, S., Quandt, T., Reich, Z., & Vujnovic, M. (2011). *Participatory journalism: Guarding open gates at online newspapers*. John Wiley & Sons.

Smith, M., Rainie, L., Shneiderman, B., & Himelboim, I. (2014). *Mapping Twitter topic networks: From polarized crowds to community clusters*. Pew.

Sustein, C. R. (2009). *Republic.com 2.0*. Princeton University Press.

Tarrow, S. (2011). *Power in movement. Social movement and contentious politics* (3rd ed.). Cambridge University Press.

Tremayne, M. (2014). Anatomy of protest in the digital era: A network analysis of Twitter and Occupy Wall Street. *Social Movement Studies*, *13*(1), 110–126.

Tremayne, M., Zheng, N., Lee, J. K., & Jeong, J. (2006). Issue publics on the web: Applying network theory to the war blogosphere. *Journal of Computer-Mediated Communication*, *12*(1), 290–310.

Tufekci, Z. (2017). *Twitter and tear gas: The power and fragility of networked protest*. Yale University Press.

Vaccari, C., Chadwick, A., & O'Loughlin, B. (2015). Dual screening the political: Media events, social media, and citizen engagement. *Journal of Communication, 65*, 1041–1061.

Van Dijck, J. (2009). Users like you? Theorizing agency in user-generated content. *Media, Culture & Society, 31*(1), 41–58.

Van Dijck, J. (2013). *The culture of connectivity: A critical history of social media.* Oxford University Press.

Van Dijck, J., & Poell, T. (2013). Understanding social media logic. *Media and Communication, 1*(1), 2–14.

Van Dijck, J., Poell, T., & De Waal, M. (2018). *The platform society: Public values in a connective world.* Oxford University Press.

Vicari, S. (2013). Public reasoning around social contention: A case study of Twitter use in the Italian mobilization for global change. *Current Sociology, 61*(4), 474–490.

Vicari, S. (2014). Networks of contention: The shape of online transnationalism in early twenty-first century social movement coalitions. *Social Movement Studies, 13*(1), 92–109.

Vicari, S. (2015). Exploring the Cuban blogosphere: Discourse networks and informal politics. *New Media & Society, 17*(9), 1492–1512.

Vicari, S. (2017). Twitter and non-elites: Interpreting power dynamics in the life story of the (#)BRCA Twitter stream. *Social Media + Society, 3*(3), 2056305117733224.

Wahl-Jorgensen, K. (2019). *Emotions, media and politics*. John Wiley & Sons.

Walker, S., Mercea, D., & Bastos, M. (2019). The disinformation landscape and the lockdown of social platforms. *Information, Communication and Society, 22*(11), 1531–1543.

Wikimedia Foundation (2020). https://wikimediafoundation.org/. Retrieved 18 June 2021.

Yang, G. (2016b). Narrative agency in Hashtag activism: The case of #BlackLivesMatter. *Media and Communication, 4* (4), 13–17.

Yardi, S., & boyd, d. (2010). Dynamic debates: An analysis of group polarization over time on Twitter. *Bulletin of Science, Technology & Society, 30*, 316–327.

Zappavigna, M. (2011). Ambient affiliation: A linguistic perspective on Twitter. *New Media & Society, 13*(5), 788–806.

3 Health Advocacy and Activism

Introduction

Health advocacy and activism encompass a range of actions and practices that aim at challenging existing health and medical policy, related politics and belief systems, and accepted and dominant ways of doing scientific research (Brown & Zavestoski, 2004, p. 679). We can think of a number of examples of such actions happening over the past two centuries. In the late 1800s and early 1900s, for instance, Black women activists advocated for social justice in health, building the basis for public health services for African Americans. In the 1960s and 1970s the women's health movement—while encouraging women's self-empowerment—began challenging medical definitions of disease, associating them with patriarchal norms detrimental to women's health. More or less in the same period anti-tobacco activist groups mobilised against smoking, and for changes in public attitudes toward smoking. Ten years later, AIDS patients advocated for clinical research that could lead to the discovery of a treatment for their disease while mental health activists marched for the rights of mentally disabled patients (Brown et al., 2010, p. 380; Cordner et al., 2014; Epstein, 1995, 1996; Zoller, 2005, p. 342). In the 1990s, breast cancer activists were first to draw public attention to the environmental causes of breast cancer (Brown et al., 2004; McCormick et al., 2003; Pezzullo, 2003), shifting the focus from individual responsibility to structural problems that increase individual risks. These and many other *health social movements* share a common element: they frame health as a political issue and, as such, an issue that deserves activist attention.

This chapter starts by offering a number of definitions relevant to health advocacy and activism both to draw a trajectory of collective actors that have contributed to the emergence of participatory cultures of health and illness—especially in relation to specific patient communities—and to review key concepts to study and understand these cultures. It then discusses the notions of illness identity, illness narrative and self-advocacy as central to the emergence of these cultures. Finally, it focuses on the concepts of experiential knowledge and lay expertise to investigate the role of different types of knowledge and expertise feeding into the participatory cultures of health and illness of the twenty-first century.

DOI: 10.4324/9780429469145-4

Health Advocacy and Activism: Definitions and Actors

Health Social Movements

Health social movements are "collective challenges to medical policy, public health policy and politics, belief systems, research and practice which include an array of formal and informal organisations, supporters, networks of co-operation and media" (Brown & Zavestoski, 2004, p. 679). In practice, the label "health social movements" works as a broad category that brings together groups mobilising for research on specific biomedical topics, advocating for widened participation in traditional decision-making around public funding of medical research, targeting environmental causes of specific diseases, advocating for new therapies, or working with private entities to develop health products (Epstein, 2008, p. 505). Overall, health social movements advocate for the inclusion of non-scientific and non-governmental views in the management of public health, in line with the idea that the contemporary "scientization of decision-making . . . can exclude the public from important policy debates and diminish public capacity to participate in the production of scientific knowledge itself" (Brown & Zavestoski, 2004, p. 681).

The "scientization" Brown and Zavestoski refer to in their work on health social movements translates in the contemporary quest for scientific evidence to inform policy making. In reality, this quest itself often constitutes a veiled attempt to conceal the politicisation of health policy making. In the coming years, for instance, we will most likely see debates on the way scientific expertise has been embedded in the management of the Covid-19 pandemic in different countries, with varying levels of transparency and success. It is not surprising, for example, that most of the daily coronavirus press conferences in the UK were held by a member of the government supported by at least one senior scientific advisor (e.g., the Chief medical officer for England (Sample & O'Carroll, 2020)). In fact, the centrality of science in arguments used to deliver the rationale for public health decision making in the UK became ever more evident when, in mid-March 2020, the government drastically changed its approach to the pandemic, enforcing restrictions on people's movement that had been defined non necessary only a few days earlier. Addressing journalists' questions on the reasons for this sudden policy U-turn, prime minister Boris Johnson said: "science has changed" (Steel, 2020).

When linked to scientific evidence, health policy foregrounds the role of scientific expertise by simultaneously downplaying that of public knowledge. In fact, a claim often advanced by health social movements is that patients' voice in the management of public health is too limited. Constraints to patients' agency are common both in traditional models of health management that exclude patients from health consultations and in paternalist approaches to patients' involvement in their health decision-making (Thompson, 2007). In practice, health activism, and patient activism more specifically, holds a twofold relationship with medicine: on one hand, they depend on medical expertise in the development of scientific research with diagnostic and prognostic objectives—on the other, they challenge the social, cultural, economic and often politicised dominance of medical authority in public health decision-making.

Drawing upon the American tradition of social movement theory, Brown and Zavestoski (2004) provide a typology of health social movements that describes three ideal types of activist actors: access movements, constituency-based movements and embodied movements. Health access movements address issues related to access to healthcare and to the provision of related services—goals typical of both traditional and more recent examples of health activism—like those mentioned at the beginning of this section. Constituency-based health movements focus on health inequalities and health inequity across social groups, with African American women' activism of the late 1800s and early 1900s offering a clear example of this. Finally, embodied health movements are grounded in personal understandings of health and illness; they mobilise for disease, disability or illness communities by countering or combining medical science with knowledge based on personal experiences. Thus, embodied health movements are characterised by three key elements: they introduce embodied experiences of health and illness in activist practices themselves, they challenge the success of medical science in solving health problems, often highlighting the way these problems are socially and economically mediated, and they enhance collaborations between patients, patients' families, health professionals and lay people via what we may call instances of fluid interaction.

Embodied movements move the boundaries "between what are considered to be patient skills and initiatives and what remains the responsibility of the doctor" (Barbot, 2006, pp. 538–539), and as such have also been labelled as "boundary movements" (Brown et al., 2004; McCormick et al., 2003): they blur traditional distinctions between lay people and professionals. These traditional boundaries are blurred via "citizen/science alliances", namely, lay-professional collaborations in which citizens and scientists work together on issues identified primarily by the former (McCormick et al., 2003, p. 547). Perhaps not surprisingly, in the emergence of these alliances, patient advocacy organisations have long played a key role.

Patient Advocacy Organisations: From Auxiliaries to Scientific Partners

While it is evident that the primary actors involved in health advocacy and activism have always been groups or organisations populated—at least in part—by patients, defining these entities and their composition is a challenging task, for heuristic and pragmatic reasons (Baggott & Forster, 2008, pp. 86–88; Chamak, 2008, p. 78; Epstein, 2016, pp. 2–3; Huyard, 2009a; Wood, 2000, pp. 21–24). In heuristic terms, different interpretations of the meaning of health care and management have made it difficult to identify a commonly agreed definition of groups advocating for health research, care, and delivery. The label "health consumer groups" (Allsop et al., 2004) for instance, has proven controversial as the use of the word "consumer" sounds misleading in relation to contexts characterised by public health systems as opposed to health insurance systems (Baggott & Forster, 2008, p. 86). On pragmatic grounds, these bodies' membership very much depends on the disease population they represent and on the participation of health professionals. Children's diseases or debilitating conditions, for instance, are by necessity in most cases advocated for by patients supported by family members or by family members alone (Chamak, 2008; Huyard, 2009a). Moreover, in many cases, organisations of this sort originate from collaborations among patients, patients' families and health professionals, with these actors playing different roles in the organisation's life and plans of action (Baggott & Forster, 2008, p. 85; Wood, 2000, pp. 21–24). All limits having been considered; I will use the term "patient advocacy organisation" to address any non-governmental organisation advocating for a disease patient community.

As Baggott and Forster show in their comparative study of EU groups, patient advocacy organisations usually originate with the aim of supporting the implementation of services for patients and their families, but they then often progressively become "more politically aware and increasingly engaged in lobbying" (2008, p. 87). Primarily drawing upon their members' lay knowledge (Allsop et al., 2004, p. 746), patient advocacy organisations turn political when they address the public arena to raise health-related issues and suggest solutions within a frame of public interest, that is, a frame that goes beyond the private illness experience. Different disease-related patient advocacy organisations are now connecting to, and influencing, one another, with political agendas that are increasingly affected by "political, cultural, and technoscientific opportunities" (Epstein, 2016, p. 7) in the context where they operate. Khan Best suggests that the effects of these agendas include "changes in the categories and meanings that shape political decision-making" (2012, p. 796). In her longitudinal study of patients' advocacy in the US, the author shows that patient advocacy organisations have been shaping political decision-making in a way to obtain direct benefits (e.g., financial support), distributive changes (e.g., more financial support for certain disease populations than others) and systemic effects (e.g., changes in the structure of decision making).

The action of patient advocacy organisations is also often associated with alternative or collaborative routes for knowledge production. The traditional division of skills between health professionals and patients—with the former holding power over medical knowledge and policy access and the latter dealing with the psychosocial aspects of illness—was overturned when patient advocacy organisations "joined established actors in the production of medical and scientific knowledge" (Barbot, 2006, p. 539). According to this new model, not only do "active patients" (Barbot, 2006) share relevant information on their illness and generate resources for self-support, they also engage in the *production* of scientific knowledge. Landzelius introduces yet another label for health social movements that directly challenge traditional boundaries between health professionals and patients, that of "'patient organisation movements': a label that clearly calls attention to the figure of the patient, the phenomenon of organisation, and the dynamics of movements" (2006, p. 530).

Landzelius' work—together with that of several scholars primarily from the field of medical sociology (see, among the others, Abma, 2006; Barbot, 2006; Caron-Flinterman et al., 2005, 2007; Epstein, 1995, 1996; Rabeharisoa, 2003, 2006)—focuses on the role of patient advocacy organisations in laying the grounds for successful interactions and bridging the gaps between patients, health professionals and health policymakers.

Patient advocacy organisations can advance different interpretations of illness, knowledge, and power relations. Barbot (2006), for instance, describes two generations of organisations mobilising for AIDS patients in France. First generation organisations, emerged at the outset of the epidemic, positioned themselves as *mediators* between AIDS sufferers and society, protecting the identity and confidentiality of their members. Second generation organisations, developing in the 1990s, instead openly defined themselves as *associations of sufferers*. Within the former model, patients were seen as managers of their own illness and in need of mediating means to connect with health professionals. Less than ten years later, within the second-generation model, patients were framed as directly involved in the development of medical and scientific knowledge. A similar point is made by Chamak (2008) in relation to French organisations advocating for autistic individuals. According to her study, third generation associations, emerging in the 1990s, have been fighting to get experiences of autism considered as knowledge that deserves the attention of public officials and professionals, and to get autistic individuals considered as partners in decision-making. In practice, they have been advocating for epistemic, political and identity changes in the public management of autism as a human condition. Similar claims have been advanced by the French associations advocating for muscular dystrophy studied by Rabeharisoa (2003), with these associations' direct engagement in research marking "partnership models" of patient advocacy organisations.

In sum, at the very least, patient advocacy organisations have now long worked towards the expansion of discursive space around specific health conditions and enhanced interactions between patients and different actors involved in biomedical research and health policy making. At the very core of these dynamics, three processes are particularly central to the study of participatory cultures of health and illness: the emergence of individual and collective illness identities, the development of different models of self-advocacy action, and the progressive recognition of patients' expertise.

Conceptual Tools to Study Participatory Cultures of Health and Illness

Illness Identity

The shifts described in the previous section imply renegotiations of our understanding and experience of being patients, patients' carers, and health experts. A number of empirical studies of health advocacy highlight how the "category of the patient" (Landzelius, 2006) often builds around interpersonal bonding and solidarity-building among sufferers, with patienthood becoming a community bond. At the heart of these bonding processes is the feeling of sharing something that is not easily understood by or communicated to those who do not experience the same condition. In other words, these community relations originate in the act of sharing common definitions of the self based on illness experiences.

Charmaz's (1991, 2002a, 2002b) work on the way individuals with chronic illnesses experience their condition as embedded in their everyday life has laid the foundation for scholarly work on "illness identities". Charmaz (1991) provides a remarkable account of the relationship between illness, time and identity, showing how any change in the development of chronic health conditions marks a shift in the patient's experience of time, with consequent renegotiations of past, present and future relationships, choices and actions—and knock-on effects on self and identity. Looking at its social dimension allows us to frame illness as a lived experience, a "biographical disruption" (Bury, 1982) that leads to searching for new meanings, for instance in the reasons behind symptoms or life expectancy. This disruption happens at the level of everyday behaviours, which are suddenly scrutinised to understand illness' causes and effects. It develops at the cognitive level, with individuals rethinking their biography. It occurs in unprecedented acts of resource mobilisation, made necessary by the presence of new challenges.

While a long line of investigation—especially in the field of cultural anthropology—has focused on the cultural roots of illness interpretations, highlighting how illness identities are heavily informed by cultural knowledge and models, less attention has been paid to the way illness identities feed into health collective action. That is, how not only personal but also collective identities are negotiated and renegotiated through illness and how these processes inform instances of health activism. If we shift the focus to collective identities in contentious politics, we reconnect with Melucci's (1995) work on collective identities as at the very core of activism (see Chapter 2). Barker (2002, p. 283) draws exactly this connection between social movement studies and sociological research of health and illness:

> public narratives help individuals formulate the claims "I am one of us", "I am not one of them"—claims that reveal how identity simultaneously exists at the individual and collective level . . . [F]ew scholars have explored the way in which illness might operate as the basis for identity construction.

In sharing personal experiences, individuals co-construct the meaning of their illness: they co-define symptoms and collectively assess treatment options. The illness communities emerging from these encounters help individuals make sense of their experiences through binding processes, with new subjectivities emerging around illness and its management. In the context of health activism, collective illness identities draw upon shared understandings and performances of the self, with illness narratives, namely stories of health and illness, providing cognitive resources to build collective action.

In her (2004) work on breast cancer activism in the San Francisco Bay Area, Klawiter looks at identity and health social movements from the opposite perspective, namely, one that focuses on how activist practices can shape illness experiences and identities. Klawiter's study shows that health activism changes the relationship with "disease regimes", namely, with the "institutionalised practices, authoritative discourses, social relations, collective identities, emotional vocabularies, visual images, public policies and regulatory actions through which diseases are socially constituted and experienced" (Klawiter, 2004, p. 851). In other words, sustained and visible health activism has the potential to alter the way a disease is addressed and framed by institutional and non-institutional actors, with a knock-on effect on understandings of the disease in both those involved in activist practices and those exposed to the language of these practices (e.g., via media coverage).

To conclude, illness experiences affect individuals' conceptions of self and identity, and the sharing of these experiences helps sufferers get together, leading to the emergence of *collective* illness identities. On one hand, these collective identities inform participatory practices around the shared illness, through self-help groups, patient organisations or other social movement entities. On the other hand, the emerging advocacy practices feed back into collective and individual illness identities in a circular and fluid process.

Illness Narratives

As seen in the previous section, narratives—and the act of storytelling—are at the centre of illness identity processes. After Bury's (1982) sociological interpretation of illness as a "biographical disruption", growing research, by both sociologists and medical professionals, has pointed to the relevance of "illness narratives" (Hydén, 1997) in coping with the life disruptions brought by disease. There is a key passage in Bury's work that has most likely bolstered this new body of research. While conceding that medicine exerts a form of social control in reorganising and reordering illness experiences, the author suggests that its coded actions and languages also provide patients with an often-welcomed element of objectivity and stability in a context marked by uncertainty. The limits, incompleteness and sometimes ambiguity of some of these codes, however, require to be supplemented by "a body of knowledge and meaning drawn from the individual's own biography" (1982, p. 179). In other words, while criticising views that see medicine as alienated from everyday illness experiences and that draw rigid divides between disease as medical terrain and illness as lay territory, Bury sheds light on patients' stories as essential to filling the gaps of medical knowledge.

As evident in Charmaz's (2002a, 2002b) work mentioned above, illness narratives are intrinsically linked with time as they connect events and symptoms along a temporal continuum within a biographical context. As Robinson (1990,

p. 1173) puts it, narratives "build up, document and order preceding events, findings and circumstances which together constitute a clear trajectory which constitutes the disease, sickness or illness". Turning illness into a personal story also allows others to comment and offer alternative interpretations based on their own life stories. This offers ways to negotiate illness meanings and associations. Hydén (1997, p. 55) identifies three main types of illness narratives based on different relationships between illness, narrative and narrator. An illness narrative can be a self-story of illness—a personal recounting of events experienced in relation to illness. But it can also be a story about someone else's illness. In this case, it will not be based on first-person memories of illness experience but on facts and events heard from or seen in others. A third form of illness narratives is where narrative—or the lack of it—is part of the illness itself, in patients who are or become unable to tell the story of their illness, for instance due to brain injuries. Hence, no matter the narrator or the subject at the centre of their plot, illness narratives enhance individual, collaborative and collective understandings of illness. In fact, among a number of other functions—e.g., constructing a coherent chain of illness events, making sense of illness, providing symbolic fabric for identity formation—narratives help transform illness into a collective phenomenon. As discussed earlier in relation to the emergence of collective illness identities as feeding into health social movements, sharing personal experiences bolsters the emergence of communitarian links among people with similar experiences of health and illness. This process of collectivisation, however, might be more difficult for individuals with conditions that are rare or more likely to affect minorities. While the characteristic of being rare may strengthen bonds among patients or sufferers, the same characteristic may make it harder for them to engage in successful activist action as their illness narratives often fail to resonate to the rest of society. In their research on AIDS patienthood in the 1990s US, Marshall and O'Keefe (1995), for instance, show that the social consequences of the disease more than private stories of suffering were given prominence in patients' illness narratives. In these accounts, the collective experience of AIDS was built on the basis of narratives of societal sufferance more than private pain.

Ultimately, according to the comprehensive body of work on the therapeutic value of storytelling (see Orgad, 2005, pp. 64–68), the telling of stories helps patients come to terms with their condition, redefine their social relations and reaffirm their sense of self (Bury, 2001). Despite the aforementioned challenges in collectivising the illness experience of disease minorities, narrative acts become ever more relevant in the case of illnesses that lack biomedical legitimacy or are labelled as rare, as in these instances, the "subjective experience of illness [is] routinely called into question, leading to social delegitimization and isolation" (Barker, 2002, p. 282). Narratives here play a bonding function and in so doing enhance the identitarian processes discussed in the previous section. Examples of these conditions are Fibromyalgia syndrome, addressed in Barker's work as an illness that lacks "organic explanation or demonstrable physiological abnormality" (2002, p. 279) or Huntington disease, a rare genetic condition discussed in Novas and Rose's (2000) work in relation to health activism. We will further discuss the peculiarity of rare disease communities in relation to participatory cultures of health and illness later in the chapter and again in Chapter 5.

Self-Advocacy

In the analysis of the evolution of the French AIDS (Barbot, 2006) and autistic (Chamak, 2008) movements we traced a change in the meaning of "active patient" from the 1980s onwards. This cognitive and factual shift turned patients from receivers of support to frontline advocates, often in partnership with traditional health stakeholders (e.g., health policymakers, scientists). As discussed in the previous section, personal experiences of health and illness contribute to the formation of illness identities at both the individual and the collective level. On one hand, they generate conceptions of self informed by the everyday coping with and understanding of symptoms, treatment options and questions about the future. On the other hand, via exposing themselves and their personal experience to others, individuals connect around common identity traits defined by the attributes of their illness. As a matter of fact, all these different processes put the self at the centre of health activist practices; they mark the steady increase of self-advocacy action that started in the 1990s. A passage of Klawiter's (1999) article on breast cancer cultures in the 1990 US sounds particularly relevant to highlight how patients' move to the frontline of health social movements has reshaped contemporary cultures of health and illness: "Unlike earlier historical moments in which cancer as a broad category had occupied center stage, this time it was breast cancer that moved to the center, and it was breast cancer survivors and activists who moved it there" (Klawiter, 1999, p. 105).

Self-advocacy is defined as the process "whereby individuals demonstrate an increased assertiveness or willingness to challenge providers or other medical authorities, and to actively participate in decision-making to ensure they receive the care and treatment they feel best meets their needs" (Martin et al., 2011, p. 178). While over the past three decades self-advocacy action has become central to health activist practices, it is important to note that its coming to prominence has not been equally smooth across social groups or illness communities. Literacy skills, for instance, are essential to inform health literacy, namely, an individual's capacity to access and process health information necessary to make health-related decisions. Literacy skills in general and health literacy in particular have been shown to be central to patients' self-advocacy and willingness to engage in participatory processes (Martin et al., 2011). Hence, social groups with the highest literacy skills are more likely than others to engage in self-advocacy.

Members of specific illness communities may also face more barriers than others to engage in frontline self-advocacy action. For instance, in his (2004) study of the Alzheimer Association in the US, Beard discusses a number of challenges preventing Alzheimer patients from speaking about their experiences as part of advocacy campaigns. Both Association views, especially those favouring biomedical aims and addressing caregivers as clients, and external factors, like public perceptions of the disease as associated with older individuals, have fed into these barriers and into paternalistic approaches to patients. Similar considerations, although in a relatively more successful context, can be drawn in relation to the British mental health movement of the early 1990s (Rogers & Pilgrim, 1991). In fact, like Alzheimer Disease, "mental illness" is more often subject to stigmatisation than other conditions because—and this is key to self-advocacy practices—the self and its manifestations cannot be easily dissociated from the disease.

In conclusion, the 1990s shift of patient engagement towards models that see patients becoming frontline advocates of their disease is indeed common across conditions and Western cultural settings. It is however important to bear in mind that this shift has not happened without encountering internal and external barriers. Some of these barriers still prevent a number of social groups and illness communities to fully engage in self-advocacy.

Experiential Knowledge, Lay Expertise, and the Credibility Game

There is an underlying assumption in the arguments presented in the previous three sections: that patients, in building new individual or collective illness identities, in narrating their own illness—while compensating medical fallacies—and in advocating for their own self, use a form of knowledge that allows and enables them to undertake these actions.

Back in 1976, sociologist Thomasina Borkman introduced the concept of "experiential knowledge" to explain knowledge dynamics within voluntary self-help groups (e.g., stutterers self-help groups). In this pivotal work, the author distinguished between "professional knowledge" and "experiential knowledge" focusing on two key elements: the type of information knowledge is based on and the attitude towards this knowledge by its holder. Professional (or expert) knowledge can be understood as knowledge acquired via traditional institutional learning. This form of knowledge is exclusive in the sense that it cannot be gained outside specialised educational and/or training settings. Those who acquire it trust the information they are exposed to in their learning process and gain credentials exactly because of the way they have grown their knowledge via a standard and widely accepted educational route. The information feeding into experiential knowledge is instead based on personal experience of and participation in relevant factual events. Borkman defines this information as "concrete, specific and commonsensical . . . and more or less representative of the experience of others who have the same problem" (1976, p. 446). Those handling this information are certain of its value and use it as truth, as they ground its validity in their personal experience of relevant facts. Accumulated experiential knowledge leads to "experiential expertise", a form of expertise that enables holders not only to understand and explain relevant issues but also to solve problems related to them. Experiential expertise is more directly associated with authority and, at least in the self-help groups investigated by Borkman, with leadership. The key point in Borkman's (1976) work is that lay self-help groups take experiential knowledge and expertise as the primary basis for decision-making.

While professional knowledge and experiential knowledge are not mutually exclusive—e.g., a professional may have direct experience of a disease that they treat in others or a patient may be professionally trained—it is not difficult to see how the relationship between the two in both clinical and non-clinical settings might prove challenging. Again, the history of French AIDS (Barbot, 2006) and autistic (Chamak, 2008) movements and the longitudinal shift in patient organisations' work and overall framing of patienthood can help us see some of the historical dynamics underlying this relationship. During their most recent phases of development, both movements have seen a coming to prominence of patients' experiential knowledge, with increasing pressure being put to get patients' voices at the centre of health research and policy decision-making. In fact, health movements in general and patient advocacy organisations in particular have always valued patients' experiential knowledge, whether to advocate for improved access to health and care services or to ensure this access is available to minorities. The real activist focus on the value and potential of patients' experiential knowledge has however emerged with what Brown and colleagues define "embodied movements" or "boundary movements", namely the activist collective actors that counter or combine medical science with knowledge based on personal experiences (Brown et al., 2004; McCormick et al., 2003) described at the beginning of this chapter.

It was Epstein's (1995) work on the US AIDS movement that somehow transferred and developed Borkman's early conceptualisations of experiential knowledge in the field of health activism. Without directly referencing Borkman's (1976) work, Epstein (1995) further discusses how the direct experience of disease, namely experiential knowledge, often leads patients to explore and/or challenge professional knowledge. In fact, while acknowledging that cancer activists, the feminist health movement and some patient self-help groups prior to the AIDS epidemic had already handled biomedical matters credibly, Epstein sees in AIDS activists the first lay "activist-experts" (1995, pp. 413–414), namely lay people engaging in activist action while and through familiarising themselves with relevant professional knowledge. Epstein provides a comprehensive picture of the way US AIDS activists turned lay experts, namely, of how they complemented their experiential knowledge acquiring credibility within the biomedical sector, overcoming the traditional science/public boundary (Gieryn, 1983). AIDS treatment activists in particular did not only base their claims and actions on their personal experience of illness, they actively engaged with the biomedical science of the disease, learning its language and subsequently getting through the doors of its institutions (Elbaz, 1992, p. 64). They acquired credibility by making themselves seen as self- representative, that is, as the legitimate voice of people with AIDS or HIV, by engaging with epistemological and moral debates—for instance in relation to trial participation criteria or experimental drug use—and by taking sides in existing debates on clinical research (Epstein, 1995, pp. 417–423).

In a recent conversation with colleagues at the University of Sheffield, after presenting some of the work discussed in this chapter, I was asked: "If we talk of lay expertise, is there such a thing as lay ignorance?" I suppose the best answer to that question would be that "lay ignorance" is our default understanding of lay potential to cope with a situation that is usually addressed via specialist, professional knowledge. In traditional settings, patients have long been framed through a "deficit model" (Kerr et al., 1998), namely, they have been considered first and foremost as recipients of specialist care, ignorant of the means and knowledge needed to apply this care. With the emergence of front-line patient activism, especially from the 1990s onwards, this framing shifted towards a public recognition of the value of patients' experience and knowledge. It is however important to note that even in cases of health activism where patients are at the frontline of action as activist experts, a hierarchy of expertise may characterise the relationships among activists themselves, with "lay experts" leading action and caring for "lay lays" (Elbaz, 1992), namely for less experienced—and less expert—activists.

In sum, the concepts of "experiential knowledge" and "lay expertise" have gradually grown in prominence within medical sociology and social movement studies interested in health activism, also drawing increasing attention to the way patients' knowledge and expertise "can be extended by scientific (bio)medical insights . . . leading to so-called 'proto-professionalism'" (Caron-Flinterman, 2005, p. 2577). Thus, two elements seem key to understanding patients' activism and participatory potential in health research and policy decision-making. On the one hand, there is patients' experience of health and illness, which produces experiential knowledge essential to understand the lived aspects of disease. This is based on patient-specific understandings of and experiences with their bodies, their illnesses, their care, and their cure. This experiential knowledge, however, is not equipped with the professional skills and practice necessary to diagnose and treat disease itself (Prior, 2003). On the other hand, there is patients' tension to familiarise themselves with professional knowledge as evidenced by studies of patients' activism, for instance Epstein's (1995) investigation of the US AIDS movement. This tension has been shown to be most prominent in specific patient communities—those dealing with diseases about which information is limited and/or hardly accessible. The following two sections will focus exactly on these communities.

Lay Expertise and the New Genetics

The past twenty years have seen the emergence of the so-called "new genetics", a body of knowledge and techniques used to investigate hereditary health conditions. In fact, pre- and post-natal genetic testing and screening have become common practices to assess the incidence of serious clinical conditions. The widening use of genetic knowledge and techniques has been followed by extensive academic debate on the public understanding of the new genetics and on the extent to which the public should be part of the wider conversation focused on, for instance, its ethical concerns (Kerr et al., 1998, p. 41). One of the key considerations emerging from this debate is that lay expertise about the new genetics varies across social groups, reaching higher levels than average among those most directly affected by hereditary conditions. In practice, research shows that "zones of relevance" (Parsons & Atkinson, 1992) and "situated understandings of medical science through intensive experiences of a specific domain" (Lambert & Rose, 1996) enhance individuals' uptake of genetic information and services. Thus, people with hereditary conditions are likely to seek and develop good understandings of genetics and genetic issues because they feel these are directly relevant to their life.

According to Novas and Rose (2000), the new genetics has led to the emergence of a set of identifying characteristics linked to genetic risk: individuals with a genetic condition become categorised as "at risk", develop "genetic responsibility" towards their family and its future and renegotiate their social relationships to accommodate their condition in their everyday practices. In fact, while one could assume that people with genetic conditions manage similar experiences to those lived by patients with chronic diseases, the hereditary aspect of genetic conditions poses different questions and additional challenges, especially in relation to family planning (Petersen, 2006). This is how and why risk, responsibility and social relations play key roles in the life of those with genetic health conditions.

According to Petersen,

> With the genetics so-called revolution gaining pace and more and more people predicted to undergo genetic testing in the future, it is crucial to consider how healthcare may utilise the experience and knowledge of those who have to deal with the everyday demands posed by a genetic condition—arguably 'the best experts'.
>
> (2006, p. 41)

This is to say that the individual at genetic risk is, perhaps more than anybody else, to "become skilled, prudent and active, an ally of the doctor, a proto-professional—and to take their own share of the responsibility for getting themselves better" (Novas & Rose, 2000, p. 489). These considerations point to the fact that the forms of subjectivity marked by genetic risk develop new relationships with expertise—relationships informing a new kind of citizenship that has been labelled as "biological-citizenship" (Rose & Novas, 2005). As a matter of fact, individuals with genetic conditions, especially rare diseases, have been shown to demand increasing participation in research, policy and care practices related to their conditions (Rabeharisoa, 2003), building relational networks that cut across different levels and types of expertise. They are also likely to connect within groups populated by individuals with similar risk, like patient or trial groups. In their analysis of support groups for people with Huntington disease, Novas and Rose (2000), for instance, argue that group members become lay experts in gaining as much knowledge as possible about the disease and applying this knowledge to themselves or to the person they care for. Most importantly: "Increasingly, those at risk constitute their own forms of expertise, through support groups for those at risk or affected" (Novas & Rose, 2000, p. 506). The key argument here is that these patient and carer groups manage to share, assess, and prioritize both experiential *and* professional information. In fact, individuals with genetic conditions often acquire technical knowledge, familiarise with scientific terminology, and self-identify as experts, especially when confronting health professionals with little or no knowledge of their specific conditions (Petersen, 2006).

In sum, patient communities forming around genetic conditions seem to epitomize the growing prominence of patients' lay expertise that started to be investigated in the mid-1990s. As mentioned above, a specific set of communities populated by individuals with genetic conditions perhaps shows the most visible use of lay expertise within participatory practices: that of rare disease patients.

Genetics, Rare Diseases, and Health Advocacy

Given the general lack of information on rare diseases, the average delay in rare disease diagnosis and the scarcity of treatments for many of these conditions, rare disease patient communities are often at the centre of debates on patients' involvement in the production of health knowledge (Rabeharisoa et al., 2014). The term "rare diseases" was first established by the 1983 US Orphan Drug Act to define a cluster of health conditions by their maximum prevalence threshold in the US: one in 1,250 people (Aymé et al., 2008; Huyard, 2009b). Similar categorisations were later adopted in the European Community, Japan, South Korea, Singapore, Taiwan and Australia (Aymé et al., 2008; Huyard, 2009b, 2009c, p. 362; Remuzzi & Garattini, 2008). In the European Community, for instance, a disease is defined as rare when it affects up to 1 in 2000 people. Most of the over 6000 rare diseases so far identified have a genetic component, are chronic and are life-threatening (Eurordis, 2021; Nord, 2021).

As a matter of fact, until the 1980s the pharmaceutical industry neglected rare disease research because it considered it not profitable. The situation changed thanks to lobbying by the rare disease community, which advocated for the implementation of specific policy to enhance the development of treatments (Aymé et al., 2008). In fact, for the past thirty years, Rare Disease Patient Organisations (RDPOs) have been "crucial for the patients and their family" (Huyard, 2009c, p. 368) by acting as "boundary movements" (Brown & Zavestoski, 2004), namely, combining lay and expert knowledge and identities. This happens, for instance, when RDPOs facilitate partnership models of engagement in biomedical research, especially when they master their own research policy and when the patients they represent become "specialist" partners (Rabeharisoa, 2003, p. 2131). Drawing upon Star and Griesemer (1989), Huyard (2009b) identifies the category itself of rare diseases as a "boundary object", that is, an object that is malleable enough to be used by different actors in their social worlds and still retain a commonly agreed identity. For patients, the use of the rare diseases category is political, as it becomes a means to merge individual diseases' small populations—while "asserting their specificities" (Rabeharisoa et al., 2014, p. 196)—into a larger group with a stronger political voice. Physicians who specialise in rare diseases see this category as relative, as to them, the size of a disease population does not influence the worthiness of their work. Finally, prior to the enforcement of the Orphan Drug Act, the pharmaceutical sector saw the rare diseases drug market as a non-profitable one. With the new regulatory environment established by the Act, the sector associated with it the possibility of innovation and niche markets (Huyard, 2009b, pp. 468–469). Hence, the boundary identity of the rare diseases category distinguishes rare diseases from other "mainstream" diseases because it meets the needs of different stakeholders and in so doing enhances collaborative processes that are much more advanced than in mainstream disease constituencies (Dalgalarrondo, 2004, as cited in Huyard, 2009b).

The conceptualisations of "boundary movement" (Brown & Zavestoski, 2004) and "boundary category of rare diseases" (Huyard, 2009b) also align with that of "evidence-based activism" advanced by Rabeharisoa et al. (2014), according to which, RDPOs elaborate, and sometimes combine, experiential knowledge and professional knowledge to mobilise different stakeholders on issues raised by patients and patients' families. In the case of 22q11 deletion syndrome, for instance, evidence brought forward by a group of concerned families prompted the exploration of potential links between the syndrome and a set of psychiatric disorders, ultimately leading to a redefinition of the syndrome itself (Rabeharisoa et al., 2014). The collaborative dimension of rare disease advocacy action is also reflected in the membership of their representative organisations. Huyard (2009a)'s research, for instance, shows that these organisations may be "pluralistic" or "monistic", depending on the number of different stakeholders populating their leading group, with pluralistic ones being more likely to perform well in their advocacy and activist action.

Rabeharisoa and colleagues (2014) describe RDPOs as engaging in two different politics: a "politics of numbers" and a "politics of singularisation", with the first receiving the most academic attention. RDPOs are usually described as attempting to mainstream rare diseases in research and development practices ("politics of numbers"). In fact, given that the first obstacle to public and private intervention in the case of rare diseases is the limited number of patients affected by each individual disease, patient organisations have started networking across patient communities, drawing attention to the overall impact of rare diseases. On the websites of the major umbrella organisations for rare diseases in the EU and the US, for instance, one reads: "Rare diseases currently affect 3.5%–5.9% of the worldwide population, an estimated 30 million people in Europe and 300 million worldwide" (Eurordis, 2021). "There are approximately 7,000 rare diseases. It's estimated that 25–30 million Americans (almost 1 in10) have rare diseases" (NORD, 2021). Therefore, rare disease patient communities are working towards building a rare disease solidarity network, to both generate support for rare disease patients and raise awareness in the general public.

Ultimately, RDPOs are representative of "embodied social movements" (Brown & Zavestoski, 2004) because they often focus on the embodied experience of a disease, challenge existing—or non-existing—medical knowledge, and pursue partnerships between patients, patients' families, health professionals, health policy-makers and lay people. The collaborative interactions among these different stakeholders are enhanced by the very essence of the institutionalised category of rare diseases and emerge in definition, membership, and action dynamics. This clearly distinguishes RDPOs as developing participatory dynamics that, more than ever before, stretch lay/expert knowledge boundaries (see Chapter 5).

Conclusion

This chapter has covered key elements to study health advocacy and activism, with a focus on research looking at its actors, targets, and achievements over the past fifty years. In particular, in the past three decades patient advocacy organisations—as central collective actors mobilising for patients' access to services and against health inequalities—have advocated for the progressive integration of patients' voices in health research and policy decision making. This work has developed with the progressive shift from auxiliary models of collaborations to concrete partnerships involving patients, families, and key stakeholders.

With the progressive emergence of patients' voices in advocacy and activist action, illness narratives have grown in prominence, not only in the private lives of individuals with health conditions but also in wider public debates about health and illness. This process has fed into the formation of collective illness identities, which are at the very heart of contemporary forms of health activism. As a matter of fact, this should not sound surprising because—as discussed in the previous chapter—identity processes have been at the core of activism practices and social movement research for a very long time. The emergence of personal and collective illness narratives and identities has also enhanced forms of self-advocacy, putting the self at the centre of health advocacy messages.

An element that is partially peculiar to health activism is its close engagement with knowledge production and its constant dealing with both fruitful intersections and antagonist clashes of lay and professional knowledge. Lay interest in professional knowledge is now evident across illness communities but reaches highest levels within communities who mostly struggle to access relevant information, treatment and services, for instance due to the rarity of their disease. In fact, it is probably within these communities that the traditional lay/science boundary is stretched the most.

But how has the gradual emergence of digital media—and their progressive integration in our everyday life—contributed to or maybe altered some of the participatory practices discussed here? The next two chapters will start addressing this question by retracing the early trajectory of digital participatory dynamics related to health and illness.

Reference List

Abma, T. A. (2006). Patients as partners in a health research agenda setting: The feasibility of a participatory methodology. *Evaluation of Health Professions*, *29*, 424–439.

Allsop, J., Jones, K., & Baggott, R. (2004). Health consumer groups in the UK: A new social movement? *Sociology of Health and Illness*, *26*(6), 737–756.

Aymé, S., Kole, A., & Graft, S. (2008). Empowerment of patients: Lessons from the rare diseases community. *Lancet*, *371*, 2048–2051.

Baggott, R., & Forster, R. (2008). Health consumer and patients' organisations in Europe: Towards a comparative analysis. *Health Expectations*, *11*, 85–94.

Barbot, J. (2006). How to build an "active" patient? The work of AIDS associations in France. *Social Science & Medicine*, *62*, 538–551.

Barker, K. (2002). Self-help literature and the making of an illness identity: The case of fibromyalgia syndrome (FMS). *Social Problems*, *49*(3), 279–300.

Beard, R. L. (2004). Advocating voice: Organisational, historical and social milieux of the Alzheimer's disease movement. *Sociology of Health & Illness*, *26*(6), 797–819.

Best, R. K. (2012). Disease politics and medical research funding: Three ways advocacy shapes policy. *American Sociological Review*, *77*(5), 780–803.

Borkman, T. (1976). Experiential knowledge: A new concept for the analysis of self-help groups. *Social Service Review*, *50*(3), 445–456.

Brown, P., Adams, C., Morello-Frosch, R., Senier, L., & Simpson, R. (2010). Health social movements. *Handbook of Medical Sociology*, *380*.

Brown, P., & Zavestoski, S. (2004). Social movements in health: An introduction. *Sociology of Health & Illness*, *26*(6), 679–694.

Brown, P., Zavestoski, S., McCormick, S., Mayer, B., Morello-Frosch, R., & Gasior Altman, R. (2004). Embodied health movements: New approaches to social movements in health. *Sociology of Health & Illness*, *26*(12), 50–80.

Bury, M. (1982). Chronic illness as biographical disruption. *Sociology of Health & Illness*, *4*(2), 167–182.

Bury, M. (2001). Illness narratives: Fact or fiction? *Sociology of Health & Illness*, *23*(3), 263–285.

Caron-Flinterman, J. F., Broerse, J. E. W., & Bunders, J. F. G. (2005). The experiential knowledge of patients: A new resource for biomedical research? *Social Science & Medicine*, *60*, 2575–2584.

Caron-Flinterman, J. F., Broerse, J. E. W., & Bunders, J. F. G. (2007). Patient partnership in decision-making on biomedical research: Changing the network. *Science Technology Human Values*, *32*, 339–368.

Chamak, B. (2008). Autism and social movements: French parents' associations and international autistic individuals' organisations. *Sociology of Health and Illness*, *30*(1), 76–96.

Charmaz, K. (1991). *Good days, bad days: The self in chronic illness and time*. Rutgers University Press.

Charmaz, K. (2002a). The self as habit: The reconstruction of self in chronic illness. *OTJR: Occupation, Participation and Health*, *22*(1_suppl), 31S–41S.

Charmaz, K. (2002b). Stories and silences: Disclosures and self in chronic illness. *Qualitative Inquiry*, *8*(3), 302–328.

Cordner, A., Brown, P., & Morello-Frosch, R. (2014). Health social movements. In *The Wiley Blackwell encyclopedia of health, illness, behavior, and society* (pp. 1115–1120). Wiley.

Dalgalarrondo, S. (2004). *Recherche clinique et innovation médicamenteuse: quelle place pour les patients et leurs représentants? Une comparaison sida, cancer et maladies rares*. Paris: Rapport pour l'Agence Nationale de Recherche sur le Sida. http://cesta.ehess.fr/document.php?id=76

Elbaz, G. (1992). *The sociology of AIDS activism: The case of ACT UP/New York, 1987–1992*. Ph.D. diss., Department of Sociology, City University of New York.

Epstein, S. (1995). The construction of lay expertise: AIDS activism and the forging of credibility in the reform of clinical trials. *Science, Technology & Human Values*, *20*(4), 408–437.

Epstein, S. (1996). *Impure science: AIDS, activism and the politics of knowledge*. University of California Press.

Epstein, S. (2008). Patient groups and health movements. *The Handbook of Science and Technology Studies*, *3*, 499–539.

Epstein, S. (2016). The politics of health mobilization in the United States: The promise and pitfalls of "disease constituencies". *Social Science & Medicine*, *165*, 246–254.

Eurordis (2021). www.eurordis.org

Gieryn, T. F. (1983). Boundary-work and the demarcation of science from non-science: Strains and interests in professional ideologies of scientists. *American Sociological Review*, *48*(6), 781–795.

Huyard, C. (2009a). Who rules rare disease associations? A framework to understand their action. *Sociology of Health & Illness*, *31*(7), 979–993.

Huyard, C. (2009b). How did uncommon disorders become "rare diseases"? History of a boundary object. *Sociology of Health & Illness*, *31*(4), 463–477.

Huyard, C. (2009c). What, if anything, is specific about having a rare disorder? Patients judgements on being ill and being rare. *Health Expectations*, *12*, 361–370.

Hydén, L. C. (1997). Illness and narrative. *Sociology of Health & Illness*, *19*(1), 48–69.

Kerr, A., Cunningham-Burley, S., & Amos, A. (1998). The new genetics and health: Mobilizing lay expertise. *Public Understanding of Science*, *7*(1), 41–60.

Klawiter, M. (1999). Racing for the cure, walking women, and toxic touring: Mapping cultures of action within the Bay Area terrain of breast cancer. *Social Problems*, *46*(1), 104–126.

Klawiter, M. (2004). Breast cancer in two regimes: The impact of social movements on illness experience. *Sociology of Health & Illness*, *26*(6), 845–874.

Lambert, H., & Rose, H. (1996). Disembodied knowledge? Making sense of medical knowledge. In *Misunderstood science? The public reconstruction of science and technology*. Cambridge University Press.

Landzelius, K. (2006). Introduction: Patient organisation movements and new metamorphoses in patienthood. *Social Science & Medicine*, *62*, 529–537.

Marshall, P. A., & O'Keefe, J. P. (1995). Medical students' first-person narratives of a patient's story of AIDS. *Social Science & Medicine*, *40*(1), 67–76.

Martin, L. T., Schonlau, M., Haas, A., Derose, K. P., Rosenfeld, L., Buka, S. L., & Rudd, R. (2011). Patient activation and advocacy: Which literacy skills matter most? *Journal of Health Communication, 16*(sup3), 177–190.

McCormick, S., Brown, P., & Zavestoski, S. (2003). The personal is scientific, the scientific is political: The public paradigm of the environmental breast cancer movement. *Sociological Forum, 18*(4), 545–576.

Melucci, A. (1995). The process of collective identity. *Social Movements and Culture, 4*, 41–63.

NORD (2021). www.rarediseases.org

Novas, C., & Rose, N. (2000). Genetic risk and the birth of the somatic individual. *Economy and Society, 29*(4), 485–513.

Orgad, S. (2005). *Storytelling online: Talking breast cancer on the Internet* (Vol. 29). Peter Lang.

Parsons, E., & Atkinson, P. (1992). Lay constructions of genetic risk. *Sociology of Health & Illness, 14*(4), 437–455.

Petersen, A. (2006). The best experts: The narratives of those who have a genetic condition. *Social Science & Medicine, 63*(1), 32–42.

Pezzullo, P. C. (2003). Resisting "national breast cancer awareness month": The rhetoric of counterpublics and their cultural performances. *Quarterly Journal of Speech, 89*(4), 345–365.

Prior, L. (2003). Belief, knowledge and expertise: The emergence of the lay expert in medical sociology. *Sociology of Health & Illness, 25*(3), 41–57.

Rabeharisoa, V. (2003). The struggle against neuromuscular diseases in France and the emergence of the "partnership model" of patient organisation. *Social Science & Medicine, 57*, 2127–2136.

Rabeharisoa, V. (2006). From representation to mediation: The shaping of collective mobilization on muscular dystrophy in France. *Social Science & Medicine, 62*, 564–576.

Rabeharisoa, V., Callon, M., Filipe, A. M., Nunes, J. A., Paterson, F., & Vergnaud, F. (2014). From "politics of numbers" to "politics of singularisation": Patients' activism and engagement in research on rare diseases in France and Portugal. *BioSocieties, 9*(2), 194–217.

Rabeharisoa, V., Moreira, T., & Akrich, M. (2014). Evidence-based activism: Patients', users' and activists' groups in knowledge society. *BioSocieties, 9*(2), 111–128. 10.1057/biosoc.2014.2.

Remuzzi, G., & Garattini, S. (2008). Rare diseases: What's next? *Lancet, 371*, 1948–1949.

Robinson, I. (1990). Personal narratives, social careers and medical courses: Analysing life trajectories in autobiographies of people with multiple sclerosis. *Social Science & Medicine, 30*(11), 1173–1186.

Rogers, A., & Pilgrim, D. (1991). "Pulling down churches": Accounting for the British mental health users' movement. *Sociology of Health & Illness, 13*(2), 129–148.

Rose, N., & Novas, C. (2005). Biological citizenship. In Ong, A. & Collier, S. (Eds.) *Global assemblages: Technology, politics and ethics as anthropological problems* (pp. 439–463). Blackwell Publishing.

Sample, I., & O'Carroll, L. (2020, March 4). Prof. Chris Whitty: The expert we need in the coronavirus crisis. *The Guardian*. www.theguardian.com/society/2020/mar/04/prof-chris-whitty-the-expert-we-need-in-the-coronavirus-crisis

Star, S. L., & Griesemer, J. R. (1989). Institutional ecology, translations' and boundary objects: Amateurs and professionals in Berkeley's Museum of Vertebrate Zoology, 1907–39. *Social Studies of Science*, *19*(3), 387–420.

Steel, M. (2020, March 19). How convenient for Boris Johnson that the science on coronavirus "changed": That way he was never wrong. *The Independent*. www.independent.co.uk/voices/coronavirus-boris-johnson-schools-cruise-restaurant-theatre-a9411961.html

Thompson, A. G. H. (2007). The meaning of patient involvement and participation in health care consultations: A taxonomy. *Social Science & Medicine*, *64*, 1297–1310.

Wood, B. (2000). *Patient power? The politics of patients' associations in Britain and America*. Open University Press.

Zoller, H. M. (2005). Health activism: Communication theory and action for social change. *Communication Theory*, *15*(4), 341–364.

Part 2

Digitised and Networked Health

4 The Rise of the "Epatient" in the Internet That Was

Introduction

On 30 January 2015, 19-year-old Harvard computer science student Elana Simon, survivor of a rare paediatric cancer, introduced the then US president Barack Obama at the White House Precision Medicine announcement.[1] Unusual as it was, Simon's opening struck right at the core of one of the central elements of contemporary debates on health care and management: patients' direct involvement in research and treatment decision-making. The Precision Medicine Initiative was presented as working toward prevention and treatment plans tailored to individuals' needs

> with a longer-term aim to generate knowledge applicable to the whole range of health and disease . . . Furthermore, the initiative taps into converging trends of increased connectivity, through social media and mobile devices, and Americans' growing desire to be active partners in medical research.
>
> (Collins & Varmus, 2015, p. 793)

The inclusion of "connectivity through mobile devices" in the presentation of the Precision Medicine Initiative talks to the ever-growing role of the digital in private and public dimensions, individual and collective contexts.

Attention to the relationship between contemporary Information and Communication Technologies (ICTs) and health care is now being drawn from across a range of disciplinary fields. On one hand, a growing body of information science, health science and clinical literature takes an instrumental approach to ICTs, primarily focusing on the affordances of digital media and communication in the context of, for instance, telemedicine, eHealth, mHealth, digital medicine and digital health. On the other hand, critical social scientific research has more recently started to shed light on the lived experience of mundane digital media and communication practices related to health and illness, especially in the context of self-care. Recent explorations have looked, for instance, at health-relevant social media uses (Lupton, 2012) or at the impact of wearables both on the management of personal health data (Lupton, 2013) and on dynamics of "soft resistance" to big data practices (Nafus & Sherman, 2014; Ruckenstein &

DOI: 10.4324/9780429469145-6

Pantzar, 2017). Chapters 6 and 7 will zoom in on these explorations and ultimately advance a series of propositions about the relationship between contemporary digital media practices and participatory cultures of health and illness. To fully understand those propositions—and the lines of inquiry from which they originate—it is however essential to first look at how ICTs have been conceptualised since the emergence of early digital media practices related to health and illness. This chapter discusses these conceptualizations through two broad paradigms, which I label "service delivery" and "epatient".

ICTs in the Traditional "Service Delivery" Paradigm

The advent of telemedicine marked the official entrance of ICTs in the realm of health and medicine. While telemedicine practices had been under development for decades, the use of the word "telemedicine" in clinical publications started its real ascent in 1993 (see Figure 4.1), with studies of the application of "telecommunications technologies to provide medical information and services" in "remote electronic clinical consultation" (Perednia & Allen, 1995, p. 483).

Initially, ICTs mainly comprised one-way and two-way television processes that allowed the exchange of data between patients and physicians. With technological development, telemedicine applications have increasingly drawn upon innovations in computer and network technologies. In the introduction to their highly cited meta-analysis of studies on patients' satisfaction with telemedicine, Mair and Whitten (2000, p. 1517) write that "There is increasing interest in the use of telemedicine as a means of healthcare delivery". In an equally cited review of clinical literature, Roine and colleagues (2001, p. 765) advance that "Telemedicine is also expected to increase the fairness and equality of the distribution of services, because the accessibility of health services, especially

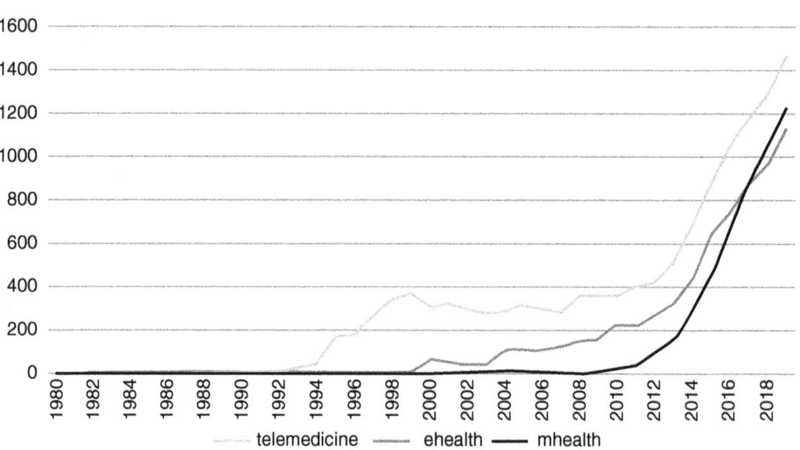

Figure 4.1 "Telemedicine", "eHealth" and "mHealth" on PubMed 1980-present.

in remote areas, can be improved". These studies suggest that the introduction of telemedicine practices was primarily framed as easing existing patient-physician relationships, with technology being used as a means to overcome geographical barriers and speed up interaction processes. These meta-analyses describe telemedicine practices as enhancing service provision and delivery, never really bolstering patients' engagement in (their) health decision-making. Even when two-way communication processes are described, as already in Perednia and Allens (1995)'s pivotal study, these are functional to deliver data from patients to physicians remotely. In the limited social science literature where telemedicine (or telehealth) is originally discussed, some concerns are advanced exactly on the general emphasis on the use of technology to simply enhance traditional patient-physician dynamics of interaction. In his 2002 editorial in the Journal of Health Communication, "Telehealth—promise or peril", Ratzan (2002, p. 257) writes: "over-emphasis on health system applications at traditional health facilities focusing on electronic medical records and related areas implies disease and clinical data mitigated by health professionals" and stresses that technology's real potential was still to be realised in the development of more personalised models of health care and management.

As a matter of fact, the early deterministic framing of technology is still very common in a bulk of interdisciplinary research that primarily sees technologies as enhancing the delivery of services from health providers to health consumers. This framing of ICTs as "conduits" (Koteyko et al., 2015) or "inert devices" (Lupton, 2012) is adopted in studies investigating at least three different digitally-enhanced patient engagement processes related to health care provision: the shortening of patient-physician physical distances, public campaigning for behavioural change and health surveillance strategies.

Technology as Shortening Physical Distances

The idea that ICTs can primarily shorten physical distances is the key rationale for the introduction of telemedicine practices but often also surfaces in the narrative produced around more recent medical practices. While telemedicine was continuing its ascent in the literature, eHealth became popular in clinical publications in 2000 while mHealth climbed up four years later, in 2004, with a dramatic acceleration in 2012 (see Figure 4.1). In 2001, Eysenbach introduced a definition of eHealth that was to become extremely popular: "an emerging field in the intersection of medical informatics, public health and business, referring to health services and information *delivered* or enhanced through the Internet and related technologies" (Eysenbach, 2001, p. 1, emphasis added). In fact, starting from the late 1990s, technology has often been described as a means to expand and enhance health-related human activities. As Oh et al. (2005: online) point out: "Most commonly, the word health was used in relation to health services delivery". According to the 51 definitions of eHealth reviewed by Oh and colleagues (2005), in technology-enhanced health processes ICTs simply ease the delivery of services from health providers to health users. Even where interaction processes are described, they are usually not controlled by patients.

The now established literature on mHealth—or the "evolution of e-health systems from traditional desktop 'telemedicine' platforms to wireless and mobile configurations" (Istepanian et al., 2004, p. 405)—often applies a similar approach to the relationship between health and (mobile) digital communication, by primarily focusing on the way via mobile devices "information and services can be delivered at appropriate times" and "penetrate into underserved or disadvantaged populations" (Whittaker et al., 2012, p. 12). Whittaker's accent on "underserved and disadvantaged populations" is representative of a common trend in mHealth—clinical and social science—literature, where technology is seen as democratising health by allowing service delivery in contexts traditionally characterised by adverse conditions.

Technology as a Means to Promote Behavioural Change

mHealth is often framed as essential to campaigns for behaviour change (Cole-Lewis & Kershaw, 2010; Fjeldsoe et al., 2009; Krishna et al., 2009; Laranjo et al., 2015; Whittaker et al., 2010). Whittaker et al. (2012, pp. 12–14), for instance, review research on the use of mHealth for smoking cessation, depression prevention, to encourage physically active lifestyles and healthful eating, to monitor mood and cognitive behavioural therapy exercises, to disseminate sexual health information and in the treatment of bulimia nervosa. Social media are often at the core of this research. Laranjo et al. (2015)'s first meta-analysis of clinical literature on social media use for health, for instance, reports a "statistically significant positive effect of [social media] interventions on behavior change, boosting encouragement for future research in this area" (p. 253). In fact, the development of apps for health promotion as part of health campaigns is now a common trend among government health bodies. As Lupton suggests, this "is an attempt to build on the popularity of such apps and to exploit their potential for recording information about an individual's exercise or dietary habits and providing constant reminders to engage in health-promoting behaviours" (2012, p. 231). Hence, in health promotional campaigns developing via mobile devices, mainstream social media platforms (see Chapter 6) and digital health platforms (see Chapter 7), lay people are often framed as addressees and recipients of centrally-controlled personalised health programmes, in many cases without participating in consultations on the use, design and policies of these programmes (Lupton, 2013, p. 267). The primary difference between traditional public health promotion campaigns and digitally-enhanced ones is that the former used public spaces to convey their messages, while the latter—via the help of digital technologies—can now directly reach more private, personal spaces (Lupton, 2012, p. 238).

Technology as Enhancing Health Surveillance

Surveillance is the third process receiving growing attention within the service delivery paradigm of health digital engagement. Chunara et al. (2013), for instance, recommend the use of Facebook's "passively generated digital data" to overcome the limits in available data around obesity. In their study of Twitter use during the H1N1 pandemic, Signorini et al. (2011, p. 6) advance: "Twitter traffic can be used not only descriptively, i.e., to track users' interest and concerns related to H1N1 influenza, but also to estimate disease activity in real time, i.e., 1–2 weeks faster than current practice allows". In their study of Facebook likes as a new source for public health surveillance, Gittelman et al. (2015, online) provide an evaluation that is representative of a common approach to social media "big data": "Online sources may provide more reliable, timely, and cost-effective . . . data than that obtainable from traditional public health surveillance systems as well as serve as an adjunct to those systems". Hence, from a surveillance perspective, social media—thanks to their widespread penetration and integration in individuals' everyday lives—are often seen as facilitating public interventions in the area of health, both for ongoing conditions like obesity (Chunara et al., 2013) and diabetes (Weitzman et al., 2011) and for crisis management, like in the case of the H1N1 pandemic (Signorini et al., 2011) and, more recently, the Covid-19 pandemic (Hou et al., 2020).

The "service delivery" paradigm of health digital engagement suggests a framing of the health-ICTs relationship in line with the traditional approach to health care and management, with health professionals holding power over medical knowledge and policy access and patients, mainly understood as health consumers, relying upon health service provision and delivery (Barbot, 2006, p. 539). Even when two-way communication processes are described, as already in Perednia and Allens (1995)'s pivotal study, these are usually framed as functional to deliver data from patients to physicians remotely. According to this view, ICT use enhances the democratisation of health and medicine by helping patients overcome inequalities in both accessing health care services and getting personalised treatments. However, these forms of digitally-enhanced patient engagement do not seem to affect the traditional top-down approach to health care and management as they ensure health care personalisation dynamics but do not challenge traditional patient-physician power relations and structures of agency.

The Rise of the "Epatient"

In 1999, American physician Tom Ferguson introduced the word "epatient" to indicate a patient that is "equipped, enabled, empowered and engaged" (Fox, 2010). Ferguson advocated for informed self-care and for a partnership model of doctor-patient relationship that would disrupt the traditional paternalistic approach to health and medicine. The epatient approach sees ICTs in general, and digital media in particular, as a means for patients' knowledge acquisition, production and exchange rather than as conduits for the delivery of health care. Technology is framed as functional to self-care, especially in health information seeking and self-monitoring dynamics. At the social level, according to the epatient paradigm, digitally-enhanced health engagement develops in the form of discourse practices that enhance social support, bottom-up knowledge creation and public debate and/or activist action.

The concept of the "epatient" assumes that digital media and infrastructures have a positive impact on individuals coping with health conditions, a sort of empowering potential that allows them to gain agency in their personal management of the condition and to join forces with others living similar experiences (see Lupton, 2013). Such interpretation is of course not exempt from critiques. Orgad (2005), for instance, highlights how patients' digital media uses are often investigated as independent of the social and cultural contexts where they take place, adding: "in describing patients' experience, this kind of research often employs terms such as 'epatients' . . . as if patients' experiences existed only in relation to their online participation" (p. 16). Orgad calls for qualitative research approaches to explore experiences and meanings in patients' lives, without departmentalising their online interactions. Orgad's own way to study individuals' digital media uses in relation to health and illness draws upon storytelling approaches. As we saw in Chapter 3, after Bury's (1982) sociological interpretation of illness as a "biographical disruption", growing research has pointed to the relevance of "illness narratives" (Hydén, 1997) in coping with the life disruptions brought by disease. The telling of stories is here seen as helping patients come to terms with their condition, redefine their social relations and reaffirm their sense of self (Bury, 2001). In fact, digital storytelling has been investigated as typical of online health-focused conversations since the early 2000s, when scholars started to draw attention to the way people share stories of health, illness and caring on the Internet in general (Hardey, 2002) or on online social spaces like blogs (Orgad, 2005), or multiuser environments (Bers, 2009) in particular. In her pivotal work on online breast cancer blogs, Orgad (2005) describes digital storytelling as the act of creating "a framework that would capture . . . multiple and scattered events . . . An attempt to produce a self-story that helps its teller and her listeners to make sense of her experience" (p. 43). While stressing on the need to go beyond deterministic positions that ascribe empowering potential to digital media practices on the basis of measurements and Internet penetration rates, Orgad's own fine-grained study unveils fascinating dynamics in online conversations about breast cancer. In her concluding remarks, she frames her study participants as individuals who "can explore and transmit their feelings and can appropriate a disembodied medium as a way to transform their life circumstances, however limited the transformation" (2005, p. 178).

Indeed, over a decade after the publication of Orgad's pivotal study of breast cancer digital storytelling, we can think of a number of additional limitations in ascribing a necessarily positive influence to digital media in the life of individuals managing health conditions. Issues related to the non-neutrality of contemporary digital media platforms, with specific reference, for instance, to dynamics linked to platformisation and datafication were discussed at length in Chapter 2. But these were not yet as evident in the "Internet that was" explored in Orgad's study. The following sections will focus on the main points brought forward by the epatient approach and consider relevant critiques in light of findings from digital media research. They will specifically focus on early practices related to online health information seeking, social support and knowledge production.

Health Information Seeking

Not surprisingly, early research embracing the epatient paradigm focused on how individuals engage in online health information seeking processes. This research strand primarily shows that users generally seek information online to make health-related decisions, to know about their future and to seek social support (Balka et al., 2010), without necessarily relying upon traditional medical expertise. The idea underlying this research strand is that by enabling individuals to access a range of informational sources about their disease, treatment options and research, digital media become a driving force to change existing conditions in the medical and health landscapes. The slogan "knowledge is power", often used within patient communities and advocacy initiatives (see, for instance, National Breast Cancer Foundation, 2019), probably provides the best representation for this stance. A series of studies conducted by the Pew Internet and American Life Project are at the heart of early conceptualisations of patients' online information seeking as empowering (Fox, 2008, 2010, 2011, for example). In 2008, Fox would write:

> It is not just the convenience that draws internet users, but the positive experiences that most people have with online research . . . The population of e-patients may have stabilized at 75% to 80% of internet users, but it is clear that broadband allows people to engage more deeply with information sources and with each other. And circumstances, such as a serious diagnosis or an important election, can kick that engagement into high gear.
>
> (online)

In the context of the Internet that was, several issues could already be raised to question the democratising potential of digital media: dynamics related to the online information overload (Dahlberg, 2007; Habermas, 2006, pp. 423–424 n. 3; Sustein, 2009), the commercialisation of online channels of information and communication (Noam, 2005; Papacharissi, 2008, pp. 235–236) and the centralisation of online information gateways (Hindman, 2009). In line with this research, health communications literature has focused on different digital divide issues (Wyatt et al., 2005), in particular the existing uneven levels of technology access that may prevent certain social groups from being able to access online health information (Gustafson et al., 2005; Hsu et al., 2005), the relevance of literacy skills to selection and acquisition of quality online information (Mackert et al., 2014; Zarcadoolas et al., 2002) and the general obstacles met when filtering reliable information due to the overload of online data (Eysenbach & Kohler, 2002). Perceived credibility of online sources has also been shown to highly differ across digital spaces, along with the relative effects of those sources on health-related behaviour (Hu & Sundar, 2010).

With these limitations having been acknowledged, health information seeking remains one of the key practices making epatients "active, informed health consumers" (Orgad, 2005, p. 15). Information seeking practices often intertwine with information *sharing* practices. The latter play a central role in dynamics of personal and social support, a second key process studied in the context of epatient literature.

Online Social Support

Studies of online support groups have been popular since the late 1990s, when virtual communities became a topical object of investigation. The type of support shared in these communities became so prominent to acquire a specific label: "computer-mediated social support" (Burrows & Nettleton, 2000). Groups of this type have long been studied as self-support groups, namely, as primarily providing social support to their members: patients and patients' relatives. Studies interested in online self-support groups investigate the impact of such groups on patients and patients' relatives, particularly on the emotional aspects of living with a disease. Research in this camp has measured, for instance, the relationship between type of disease and the likelihood for a patient to use online groups of support (Owen et al., 2010) or investigated the importance of online tie support (Cohen & Raymond, 2011; Wright et al., 2010). Eysenbach et al. define these groups as "mental health and social support interventions" (2004, p. 1166). In general, this work tends to investigate the extent to which online support groups enhance bridging and bonding dynamics (Putnam, 2000) across and within patient communities and how these dynamics may affect an individual's wellbeing, primarily by providing social support.

In her detailed investigation of a cancer support forum, Bambina (2007) provides a very good example of an early online support group study. She identifies three specific forms of social support characterising this and similar online support groups: emotional, informative and companionship. Emotional support is described as sentimental and affective in nature: it confers empathy and sympathy in interactions often initiated with hidden or explicit requests for support in difficult circumstances. Informational support is practical in nature, often initiated with direct requests for advice or referrals or questions on practical concerns related to coping with a condition. Chatting and humour make for the key content shared in these groups that provides a sense of companionship, through the feeling of being connected to others and part of something bigger than oneself. Bambina spends a great deal of her work explaining how these different categories intertwine with one another and how subcategories of support differently feed each one of them. While this categorisation per se might sound questionable as not conveying much of the experience of participating in and belonging to the group, let alone of the participants' wider experience of health and illness (Orgad, 2005), it does help us see how support group membership can be framed as empowering if not else for enhancing interactive channels of communication that can generate networks of social support.

Information seeking dynamics and social support intertwine with a third process that has perhaps received less attention in early epatient research but is very central to patients' agency: knowledge production and co-production.

Knowledge Production

In 2002, Hardey would write: "home pages constitute the emergence of a new genre that forms part of a broader reconfiguration of the relationship between lay and medical expertise" (p. 31). In his investigation of personal homepages providing accounts of illness experiences, Hardey identifies yet again a reconfiguration of the relationship between patients and medical and health expertise. He advances a typology of homepages based on the information shared by the authors and foregrounds the way non-medical advice becomes a core element across all types. Hardey's study seems to suggest that the Internet that was, then, did contribute to and perhaps enhance the processes we discussed in Chapter 3 in relation to the emergence of new forms of lay expertise around health and illness.

Akrich (2010) takes Hardey's research one step further in the direction of understanding the role of online health conversations—in her case, mailing lists—in the construction of health knowledge. Drawing upon literature on situated learning, Akrich's argument develops from the concept of "community of practice" (CoP), namely one that focuses on "colocated or distributed" groups (Wenger et al., 2002, p. 25) whose "participants share understandings concerning what they are doing and what that means in their lives and for their communities" (Lave & Wenger, 1991, p. 98). According to Akrich, individuals joining health-focused mailing lists form "communities of experience"; that is, CoPs specifically defined by their members' (1) interactions around their experience—in this case, of health and illness—and (2) willingness to share the said experience with others. In the course of these interactions, individual experiential information—that is, disorganised fragments of personal experience—turns into experiential knowledge, namely organic and reflective accounts of health and illness, that often combine with medical data.

As we saw in Chapter 3, experiential knowledge is clearly distinguished from expert (or professional) knowledge because, contrary to the latter, its access is not "limited to those who have met the requirements of specialised education and formal training in a discipline and who possess appropriate credentials" (e.g. medical doctors) (Borkman, 1976, p. 447). In other words, while expert knowledge is grounded in specialist education, experiential knowledge is based on personal experience. According to Akrich (2010), experiential knowledge exchanges can ultimately lead to the emergence of "epistemic communities", that is, communities sharing resources—based on the combination of (patients') experiential knowledge and (medical) expert knowledge—that are more likely to influence health policing than those based on experiential information alone (also see Haas, 1992, p. 3). In the author's words, there is a "tipping point between communities of experience and epistemic communities, that is, the point where the learning achieved within the lists, the accumulated facts, the experiential and built-up knowledge could become a form of political action" (Akrich, 2010: online). The political action Akrich refers to consists of advocacy and activism for patients' rights to health services, information and research. In practice, according to Akrich, the epistemic communities emerging from the health mailing lists analysed in her work could and did lead to the formation of patient and carer advocacy organisations or groups mobilising for patient communities.

In line with Akrich's (2010) work, Bellander and Landqvist (2020) show that patients' and carers' health blogs and forum discussions also lead to the emergence of epistemic dynamics. In particular, the authors identify epistemic dynamics in the way traditional expert knowledge is absorbed, confronted and used by those traditionally defined as lay people (e.g. patients, patients' families), namely individuals with no medical training who draw "on their experiences of illness and recovery to recommend health treatments" (Hardey, 2002, p. 41). To be clear, the epistemic dimension described in Akrich's (2010) and even more in Bellander and Landqvist's (2020) work does not translate into direct *political* action but rather into discursive practices that, by incorporating the experiential and the expert, show heightened potential to develop into health campaigning and/or advocacy.

Conclusion

This chapter has provided an overview of research and findings related to early conceptualisations of ICTs and digital practices connected to health and illness. According to what we have addressed here as the "service delivery paradigm", technology in general—and ICTs in particular—can enhance the delivery of health services from providers to consumers. We have seen that this framing is particularly common in initiatives primarily interested in shortening patient-physician *physical* distances, enhancing public campaigning for behavioural change and strengthening health surveillance strategies. While this approach certainly highlights technological potential, it tends to skim over the impact of social and personal factors on user practices and it sees patients primarily as service consumers or receivers. Even in interpretations stressing the need for interactional or participatory settings, it would be hard to identify a partnership model of patient-doctor relationship, that is, one where "active patients" (Barbot, 2006) are engaged, for instance, in the production of scientific knowledge (see Chapter 3).

While ICTs progressively entered the clinical literature very much in line with the service delivery framing, alternative conceptualisations emerged, especially among patients themselves and in social scientific research. In what we have broadly defined as the "epatient paradigm", online platforms enable patients to be more directly engaged with their self-care and in the care of others, individually and collectively—in particular, with information seeking practices, social and peer support networks and knowledge co-production. As we have seen in this chapter, these processes have much in common with the recent developments in health activism that have seen the strengthening of messages advocating for patients' direct participation in health policy and research decision-making.

The next chapter will progress on the technological trajectory started here to discuss how contemporary digital transformations have developed from the early technological models primarily addressed in this chapter (i.e., mailing lists, online forums, blogs) and progressively shaped contemporary participatory cultures of health and illness.

Note

1. The recording of the event is available at: www.youtube.com/watch?v=MKiw7yAqqsU.

Reference List

Akrich, M. (2010). From communities of practice to epistemic communities: Health mobilizations on the internet. *Sociological Research Online*, *15*(2), 1–17.

Balka, E., Krueger, G., Holmes, B. J., & Stephen, J. E. (2010). Situating internet use: Information-seeking among young women with breast cancer. *Journal of Computer-Mediated Communication*, *15*(3), 389–411.

Bambina, A. (2007). *Online social support: The interplay of social networks and computer-mediated communication*. Cambria Press.

Barbot, J. (2006). How to build an "active" patient? The work of AIDS associations in France. *Social Science & Medicine*, *62*, 538–551.

Bellander, T., & Landqvist, M. (2020). Becoming the expert constructing health knowledge in epistemic communities online. *Information, Communication & Society*, *23*(4), 507–522.

Bers, M. U. (2009). New media for new organs: A virtual community for paediatric post-transplant patients. *Convergence*, *15*(4), 462–469.

Borkman, T. (1976). Experiential knowledge: A new concept for the analysis of self-help groups. *Social Service Review*, *50*(3), 445–456.

Burrows, R., & Nettleton, S. (2000). Virtual community care? Social policy and the emergence of computer mediated social support. *Information, Communication and Society*, *3*(1), 95–121.

Bury, M. (1982). Chronic illness as biographical disruption. *Sociology of Health & Illness*, *4*(2), 167–182.

Bury, M. (2001). Illness narratives: Fact or fiction? *Sociology of Health & Illness*, *23*(3), 263–285.

Chunara, R., Bouton, L., Ayers, J. W., & Brownstein, J. S. (2013). Assessing the online social environment for surveillance of obesity prevalence. *PLoS One*, *8*(4), e61373.

Cohen, J. H., & Raymond, J. M. (2011). How the internet is giving birth (to) a new social order. *Information, Communication & Society*, *14*(6), 937–957.

Cole-Lewis, H., & Kershaw, T. (2010). Text messaging as a tool for behaviour change in disease prevention and management. *Epidemiologic Reviews*, *32*(1), 56–69.

Collins, F. S., & Varmus, H. (2015). A new initiative on precision medicine. *The New England Journal of Medicine*, *372*, 793–795.

Dahlberg, L. (2007). Rethinking the fragmentation of the cyberpublic: From consensus to contestation. *New Media & Society*, *9*(5), 827–847.

Eysenbach, G. (2001). What is e-health? *Journal of Medical Internet Research*, *3*(2), e20.

Eysenbach, G., & Kohler, C. (2002). How do consumers search for and appraise health information on the world wide web? Qualitative study using focus groups usability tests and in-depth interviews. *BMJ*, *324*(7337), 573–577.

Eysenbach, G., Powell, J., Englesakis, M., Rizo, C., & Stern, A. (2004). Health related virtual communities and electronic support groups: Systematic review of the effects of online peer to peer interactions. *BMJ*, *328*, 1166.

Fjeldsoe, B. S., Marshall, A. L., & Miller, Y. D. (2009). Behavior change interventions delivered by mobile telephone short-message service. *American Journal of Preventive Medicine*, *36*(2), 165–173.

Fox, S. (2008). The engaged E-patient population. *Pew Internet & American Life Project*. www.pewinternet.org/2008/08/26/the-engaged-e-patient-population/

Fox, S. (2010). E-patients, cyberchondriacs, and why we should stop calling names. *Pew Internet & American Life Project*. www.pewinternet.org/2010/08/30/e-patients-cyberchondriacs-and-why-we-should-stop-calling-names/

Fox, S. (2011). Peer-to-peer healthcare: Many people: Especially those living with chronic or rare diseases: Use online connections to supplement professional medical advice. *Pew Internet & American Life Project*. www.pewinternet.org/files/oldmedia//Files/Reports/2011/Pew_P2PHealthcare_2011.pdf

Gittelman, S., Lange, V., Crawford, C. A. G., Okoro, C. A., Lieb, E., Dhingra, S. S., & Trimarchi, E. (2015). A new source of data for public health surveillance: Facebook likes. *Journal of Medical Internet Research*, *17*(4), e98.

Gustafson, D. H., McTavish, F. M., Stengle, W., Ballard, D., Jones, E., Julesberg, K., . . . Hawkins, R. (2005). Reducing the digital divide for low-income women with breast cancer: A feasibility study of a population-based intervention. *Journal of Health Communication*, *10*(S1), 173–193.

Haas, P. M. (1992). Introduction: Epistemic communities and international policy coordination. *International Organization*, 1–35.

Habermas, J. (2006). Political communication in media society: Does democracy still enjoy an epistemic dimension? The impact of normative theory on empirical research. *Communication Theory*, *16*, 411–426.

Hardey, M. (2002). "The story of my illness": Personal accounts of illness on the Internet. *Health*, *6*(1), 31–46.

Hindman, M. (2009). *The myth of digital democracy*. Princeton University Press.

Hou, Z., Du, F., Jiang, H., Zhou, X., & Lin, L. (2020, March 6). Assessment of public attention, risk perception, emotional and behavioural responses to the COVID-19 outbreak: Social media surveillance in China. *Social Media Surveillance in China*.

Hsu, J., Huang, J., Kinsman, J., Fireman, B., Miller, R., Selby, J., & Ortiz, E. (2005). Use of e-health services between 1999 and 2002: A growing digital divide. *Journal of the American Medical Informatics Association*, *12*(2), 164–171.

Hu, Y., & Shyam Sundar, S. (2010). Effects of online health sources on credibility and behavioral intentions. *Communication Research*, *37*(1), 105–132.

Hydén, L. C. (1997). Illness and narrative. *Sociology of Health & Illness*, *19*(1), 48–69.

Istepanian, R. S. H., Jovanov, E., & Zhang, Y. T. (2004). Guest editorial introduction to the special section on m-health: Beyond seamless mobility and global wireless health-care connectivity information technology in biomedicine. *IEEE Transactions on Information Technology in Biomedicine*, *8*(4), 405–414.

Koteyko, N., Hunt, D., & Gunter, B. (2015). Expectations in the field of the Internet and health: An analysis of claims about social networking sites in clinical literature. *Sociology of Health & Illness*, *37*(3), 468–484.

Krishna, S., Boren, S. A., & Balas, E. A. (2009). Healthcare via cell phones: A systematic review. *Telemedicine and e-Health*, *15*(3), 231–240.

Laranjo, L., Arguel, A., Neves, A. L., Gallagher, A. M., Kaplan, R., Mortimer, N., . . . Lau, A. Y. (2015). The influence of social networking sites on health behavior change: A systematic review and meta-analysis. *Journal of the American Medical Informatics Association*, *22*(1), 243–256.

Lave, J., & Wenger, E. (1991). *Situated learning: Legitimate peripheral participation*. Cambridge University Press.

Lupton, D. (2012). M-health and health promotion: The digital cyborg and surveillance society. *Social Theory & Health*, *10*(3), 229–244.

Lupton, D. (2013). The digitally engaged patient: Self-monitoring and self-care in the digital health era. *Social Theory & Health*, *11*(3), 256–270.

Mackert, M., Champlin, S. E., Holton, A., Muñoz, I. I., & Damásio, M. J. (2014). eHealth and health literacy: A research methodology review. *Journal of Computer-Mediated Communication*, *19*(3), 516–528.

Mair, F., & Whitten, P. (2000). Systematic review of studies of patient satisfaction with telemedicine. *BMJ*, *320*(7248), 1517–1520.

Nafus, D., & Sherman, J. (2014). Big data, big questions| this one does not go up to 11: The quantified self movement as an alternative big data practice. *International Journal of Communication*, *8*, 11.

National Breast Cancer Foundation (2019, 16 October). *Knowledge is power: How to stay informed this breast cancer awareness month*. www.nationalbreastcancer.org/blog/knowledge-is-power-how-to-stay-informed-this-breast-cancer-awareness-month/

Noam, E. M. (2005). Why the Internet is bad for democracy. *Communications of the ACM*, *48*(10), 57–58.

Oh, H., Rizo, C., Enkin, M., & Jadad, A. (2005). What is eHealth (3): A systematic review of published definitions. *Journal of Medical Internet Research*, *7*(1), e110.

Orgad, S. (2005). *Storytelling online*. Peter Lang.

Owen, J. E., Boxley, L., Goldstein, M. S., Lee, J. H., Breen, N., & Rowland, J. H. (2010). Use of health-related online support groups: Population data from the California health interview survey complementary and alternative medicine study. *Journal of Computer-Mediated Communication*, *15*(3), 427–446.

Papacharissi, Z. (2008). The virtual sphere 2.0: The Internet, the public sphere, and beyond. In *Routledge handbook of Internet politics* (pp. 246–261). Routledge.

Perednia, D. A., & Allen, A. (1995). Telemedicine technology and clinical applications. *Jama*, *273*(6), 483–488.

Putnam, R. D. (2000). *Bowling alone*. Free Press.

Ratzan, S. C. (2002). Telehealth: Promise or peril? *Journal of Health Communication, 7*, 257–258.

Roine, R., Ohinmaa, A., & Hailey, D. (2001). Assessing telemedicine: A systematic review of the literature. *CMAJ, 165*(6), 765–771.

Ruckenstein, M., & Pantzar, M. (2017). Beyond the quantified self: Thematic exploration of a dataistic paradigm. *New Media & Society, 19*(3), 401–418.

Signorini, A., Segre, A. M., & Polgreen, P. M. (2011). The use of Twitter to track levels of disease activity and public concern in the US during the influenza A H1N1 pandemic. *PLoS One, 6*(5), e19467.

Sustein, C. R. (2009). *Republic.com 2.0*. Princeton University Press.

Weitzman, E. R., Adida, B., Kelemen, S., & Mandl, K. D. (2011). Sharing data for public health research by members of an international online diabetes social network. *PLoS One, 6*(4), e19256.

Wenger, E., McDermott, R. A., & Snyder, W. (2002). *Cultivating communities of practice: A guide to managing knowledge*. Harvard Business Press.

Whittaker, R., Borland, R., Bullen, C., Lin, R. B., McRobbie, H., & Rodgers, A. (2010). Mobile phone-based interventions for smoking cessation. *Sao Paulo Medical Journal, 128*(2), 106–107.

Whittaker, R., Merry, S., Dorey, E., & Maddison, R. (2012). A development and evaluation process for mHealth interventions: Examples from New Zealand. *Journal of Health Communication, 17*(sup1), 11–21.

Wright, K. B., Rains, S., & Banas, J. (2010). Weak-tie support network preference and perceived life stress among participants in health-related, computer-mediated support groups. *Journal of Computer-Mediated Communication, 15*(4), 606–624.

Wyatt, S., Henwood, F., Hart, A., & Smith, J. (2005). The digital divide, health information and everyday life. *New Media & Society, 7*(2), 199–218.

Zarcadoolas, C., Blanco, M., Boyer, J. F., & Pleasant, A. (2002). Unweaving the web: An exploratory study of low-literate adults' navigation skills on the World Wide Web. *Journal of Health Communication, 7*(4), 309–324.

5 From Patient Organisations to Patient Networks

Introduction

As seen in Chapter 3, advocacy actors and patient groups have long been central to health advocacy and activism (Epstein, 2007; Landzelius, 2006). For the past thirty years, scholars have described a progressive increase in the number of collective actors representing specific patient communities (Allsop et al., 2004, p. 741; Epstein, 2007, p. 500) and with it the enhanced public visibility of health activism advocating for participatory cultures of health and illness. However, the digital dimension of these dynamics has so far remained underexplored. A relevant contribution has recently been advanced by Petersen and colleagues (2019) who, building on work by Rabinow (1992) and Rose and Novas (2005), have introduced the concept of "bio-digital citizenship" to address the way in which digital media have progressively shaped health advocacy with a new orientation towards prioritising publicity and funding over other goals. By drawing initial connections between the literature on digital media, participation and citizenship covered in Chapter 2 and the work on health advocacy and activism discussed in Chapter 3, this chapter talks to this emerging literature by discussing the affordances of digital media and communication for patient advocacy organisations.

As part of the shift towards visible forms of health advocacy, a specific category of patient-centred organisations started growing towards the end of the 1980s, when several uncommon diseases for the first time were collectively defined under the label of "rare diseases" (see Chapter 3). While contemporary research on the activity of organisations advocating for rare disease patients—including a range of comparative studies (Huyard, 2009a, 2009b, 2009c; Rabeharisoa, 2003, 2006; Rabeharisoa et al., 2014a)—is slowly growing, we still know very little about how these organisations exploit digital communication platforms to introduce themselves, frame their identity as advocacy actors and engage publics in the production and sharing of health information. In this chapter, I address this lacuna by drawing upon work that Franco Cappai and I carried out in 2016 within a research project focusing on rare disease patient organisations.

The chapter starts by discussing how patient organisations advocating for rare diseases use their institutional websites to present themselves as engaging

DOI: 10.4324/9780429469145-7

with different forms of collective action and interacting with a range of stakeholders. This is functional to present a typology of rare disease patient organisations based on official online self-presentation practices. Drawing upon Bennett and Segerberg's (2013) work on the "logic of connective action" and on digital media work interested in the emergence of personalised and crowdsourced forms of activism and public engagement (e.g., Papacharissi, 2015) (see Chapter 2), the remainder of the paper specifically focuses on the digital mechanisms embedded in these organisation websites. This is functional to assess the extent to which these mechanisms offer individualised forms of public engagement and alternative informational pathways for rare disease patient communities, and eventually enhance participatory practices.

Ultimately, this chapter follows the digital trajectory initiated in Chapter 4 and takes us one step closer to understand the role of digital media platforms in contemporary participatory cultures of health and illness.

Rare Disease Advocacy

As mentioned earlier, rare disease patients face extremely adverse conditions, primarily because of the lack of information and knowledge on their disease in both the medical community and the general public. Perhaps not surprisingly, research into the digital practices of people with rare diseases shows that they are more likely than others to look for peers online, primarily given the general lack of information and knowledge relevant to their disease: "People living with a rare disease, their own or a loved one's, have honed their searching, learning, and sharing skills to a fine point. They endlessly scan resources for clues to try to cope with and mitigate the inevitable complications and setbacks that come from rare diseases" (Fox, 2011).

Patient organisations have always played an extremely important role for rare disease patients, for instance, by lobbying for the implementation of specific policy to incentivise the development of treatments for rare diseases, playing a pivotal role in the development of treatments themselves (Aymé et al., 2008), and helping patients find each other despite the rarity of their conditions. Given the relevance of online sources for rare disease patients and their families, and the mediating role of advocacy organisations, official organisation websites have traditionally represented an extremely important public dimension for rare disease patient groups.

In 2016, Franco Cappai and I investigated the website presence of a number of international rare disease patient organisations. We wanted to explore how these organisations construct their identity online and how the digital mechanisms (i.e. various more or less interactive website elements) studied by Bennett and Segerberg (2013) in relation to contemporary digital activism (see Chapter 2) related to rare disease advocacy. We selected the rare diseases to be included in our study on the basis of their receiving recent approvals for treatments by the EU and US regulatory authorities (i.e., European Medicine Agency (EMA) and Food and Drug Administration (FDA), respectively).

Given that rare disease patient organisations have historically been involved in partnership models of research development (Rabeharisoa, 2003), we took treatment approval as an indicator that patient organisations representing the relevant diseases were likely to be active in lobbying and advocacy action. We identified the online top-ranked organisation websites advocating for the chosen diseases to isolate the patient organisations that were strategically exploiting online information politics. We included all the organisations appearing in the Google.com list of the first 10 retrieved webpages (see Table 5.1).

The following sections first discuss the way rare disease patient organisations define and build advocacy actions via their official websites and then focus more specifically on the role of the digital mechanisms embedded in this online presence in terms of enhancing specific forms of connective action.

Table 5.1 Rare disease and patients' advocacy organisations.

Rare disease	*Patient organisation*	*Location*	*Website address*
Addison's Disease	Addison's Disease Self Help Group	UK	www.addisons.org.uk
Amyloidosis	Amyloidosis Foundation	US	www.amyloidosis.org
Ataxia	Ataxia UK	UK	www.ataxia.org.uk
Blood Cancer	Leukaemia & Lymphoma research	UK	leukaemialymphomaresearch.org.uk
Childhood Auto Inflammatory Disease	Stop CAID Now	US	www.stopcaidnow.org
Childhood Cancer	Children with Cancer UK	UK	www.childrenwithcancer.org.uk
Chronic Lymphocytic Leukaemia (CLL)	CLL Support Association	UK	www.cllsupport.org.uk
Chronic Myelogenous Leukemia (CML)	The National CML Society	UK	www.nationalcmlsociety.org
Cryopyrin-Associated Periodic Syndromes (CAPS)	Nomid Alliance	US	www.nomidalliance.org
Cystic Fibrosis	Cystic Fibrosis Trust	UK	www.cysticfibrosis.org.uk
Cystic Fibrosis	Cystic Fibrosis Canada	Canada	www.cysticfibrosis.ca
Cystic Fibrosis	Cystic Fibrosis Foundation	US	www.cff.org
Friedreich's Ataxia	FARA	US	www.curefa.org
Gaucher Disease	Gaucher Association	UK	www.gaucher.org.uk
Gaucher Disease	National Gaucher Foundation, Inc.	US	www.gaucherdisease.org
Hereditary Angioedema	US Hereditary Angioedema Association (HAEA)	US	www.haea.org

(*Continued*)

Table 5.1 (Continued)

Rare disease	*Patient organisation*	*Location*	*Website address*
Hereditary Angioedema	HAEUK	UK	www.haeuk.org
Idiopathic Pulmonary Fibrosis	Pulmonary Fibrosis Foundation	US	hwww.pulmonaryfibrosis.org
Leukaemia	Leukaemia Foundation	Australia	www.leukaemia.org.au
Lymphoma	Lymphoma Research Foundation	US	www.lymphoma.org
Lynch Syndrome	Lynch Syndrome International	US	www.lynchcancers.com/
Multiple Myeloma	Multiple Myeloma Research Foundation	US	www.themmrf.org
Myeloma	International Myeloma Foundation	US	myeloma.org
Myeloma	Myeloma UK	UK	www.myeloma.org.uk
Myeloproliferative neoplasms	MPN Research Foundation	US	www.mpnresearchfoundation.org
Pituitary Disease	The Pituitary Society	US	www.pituitarysociety.org
Pulmonary Fibrosis	Coalition for Pulmonary Fibrosis	US	www.coalitionforpf.org
Short Bowel Syndrome	Short Bowel Support (SBS)	US	www.shortbowelsupport.com
Short Bowel Syndrome	Short Bowel Syndrome Foundation	US	www.shortbowelfoundation.org
Tuberous Sclerosis	Tuberous Sclerosis Alliance	US	www.tsalliance.org
Tuberous Sclerosis	Tuberous Sclerosis Association	UK	www.tuberous-sclerosis.org

Patient Organisation Websites as Means to Build Identity and Action

Establishing the Identity of Rare Disease Patient Advocacy

The organisations in our study covered a long history of rare disease patient advocacy, with the oldest being the Cystic Fibrosis Foundation, established in the US in 1955, and the youngest being the National CML Society and the Short Bowel Syndrome Foundation, both founded in the US in 2010. The remaining organisations originated sometime between these two time points, with more than two thirds of them being born after the enforcement of the

US Orphan Drug Act in 1983. As a matter of fact, evidence from previous research shows that patient advocacy organisations and groups across illness communities have kept increasing starting from the early 1980s (Allsop et al., 2004, p. 741). Allsop and colleagues link this trend with the need to cope with the "biographical disruption" (Bury, 1982) brought by the experience of living or caring for someone with a health condition and engaging with a range of forms of action. When it comes to rare disease illness communities, this need combines with that of finding the rare others with the same conditions and sharing the scarce available information about the condition itself.

To investigate the way our sample organisations constructed their identity via their official websites, we focused on the narratives they used to describe how and why they were founded (see Table 5.2).

Most of the organisations in our study were founded by individual stakeholders—patients alone or with families. Collaborations between patients and health professionals were rarely mentioned as leading to the formation of an organisation. This suggests that, despite the fact that pluralistic organisations have been described as achieving better and faster results than monistic ones (Huyard, 2009a), rare disease patient organisations are still often founded for the will of, and by, patients and their families rather than out of boundary collaborations with health professionals. Only on the websites of organisations advocating for Friedreich's Ataxia patients, were health professionals part of the organisation's birth narrative, possibly suggesting that the characteristics of a rare disease may influence the presence or absence of boundary collaborations prior to the emergence of an advocacy organisation:

> FARA was founded in September 1998 by a group of patient families and three of the world's leading FA scientists—Drs Rob Wilson, Bronya Keats, and Massimo Pandolfo.
>
> (FARA, 2016)

Table 5.2 The identity of rare disease patients' advocacy organisations.

Identity
1. Founders
a. Patients (and/or families) and physicians
b. Patients' parents or families only
c. Patients only
2. Reasons to be
a. To improve knowledge in general practitioners
b. To provide exclusive support for a specific patient community
c. To support research through fundraising
d. To find a cure
e. To help patients and families
f. To give a voice to the community
g. To provide support internal to the community
h. To raise awareness

> Ataxia UK began life modestly back in 1963, when Dr R L Hewer and Dr Norman Robinson ('Robbie') encouraged a group of parents whose children had Friedreich ataxia to get together for mutual support.
>
> (Ataxia UK, 2016)

When the rationale behind the foundation was clearly phrased in the organisations' websites, in most cases it centred on the aim to help patients and their families, primarily by providing bonding material and emotional support for their rare disease community. Recognition claiming also played a central role (Huyard, 2009a), especially for extremely rare diseases. In these cases, support was explicitly described as in the form of providing a "voice" to the community. In fact, some of the organisations stressed on the exclusivity of the patient community they represented and framed both the identity of the community and the nature of their work as unique (Best, 2012, p. 794; Huyard, 2009c, p. 362; Rabeharisoa et al., 2014b). Supporting research and raising awareness among both physicians and the general public were the remaining most likely purposes mentioned in foundation narratives. In particular, the former was sometimes framed with explicit reference to the potential of fundraising activities to enhance research funding, other times with a bolder focus on the organisation's potential agency in contributing to "finding a cure".

In sum, no matter the life-span of a rare disease patient organisation, patients' and families' experiences of a rare disease appeared to be a core narrative element both in delivering their "what we are" and in providing a strong identity component in framing their collective advocacy. In fact, while community support, scientific advancement and recognition claiming were core objectives in the reason-to-be of these organisations, health professionals were not central, and policymakers were totally absent.

Defining the Areas of Action of Rare Disease Patient Advocacy

The narratives of action provided on the organisation websites centred on four general themes: providing services for patients and families, enhancing scientific advancement, raising awareness in the general public and impacting policymaking (see Table 5.3).

Providing Services for Patients and Families

All the sample organisations reported on their traditional role as service providers for patients and their families. While this may not be extremely surprising, the weight given to different specific activities pertaining to this role provides an interesting insight into the definition of peer-support in rare disease patient communities. In fact, for all of the sample organisations, a central service was grounded in information sharing activities, with these being patient newsletters, events (e.g.,

Table 5.3 The areas of action of rare disease patients' advocacy organisations.

Action
1. Providing services for patients and families
a. Counselling support
b. Helpline
c. Financial support
d. Funding accommodation services
e. Funding medical services
f. Grants for patients and families
g. Information
2. Enhancing scientific advancement
a. Research funding
b. Research career development awards
c. Organisation of/Contribution to clinical trials
d. Organisation of/Contribution to research projects
e. Organisation of/Contribution to research programmes
f. Boundary information sharing
3. Raising awareness in the general public
a. Billboard
b. Conference
c. News presence
d. Awareness day or month
e. YouTube video
f. Fundraising activities
4. Impacting policy making
a. Work to diminish bureaucracy around clinical trials
b. Contribution to policy
c. Monitoring of policy making
d. Work to improve screening programmes
e. Work to increase or save public funding
f. Work to raise awareness with policy makers

meetings, community workshops, conferences), technology-enhanced informational tools (e.g., additional websites, webcasts, webcast libraries, helplines), educational tools in general (e.g., factsheets, consensus documents, information packs, scientific publications) and counselling services. This seems to reframe peer-support as a way to enhance knowledge within the patient community, hence shifting the attention from the traditional focus on emotional peer-support to a redefinition of rational and crowdsourced community agency.

The financial support provided by these organisations may come in the form of grants or funding for medical or accommodation services, also depending on the organisation's size, history, and financial resources. Community support via service delivery was framed along the binary line of enhancing the availability of information and financial resources, to increase awareness and knowledge building on one hand and increase patients' quality of life on the other.

Enhancing Scientific Advancement

If the delivery of services for patients and their families, traditionally considered as the primary role for patient advocacy organisations (Baggott & Forster, 2008), appeared as a central area of action across our sample, evidence also showed that rare disease organisations equally value the importance of their active contribution to scientific advancement. Given the general lack of information and scientific knowledge relevant to rare disease diagnosis and treatment (Huyard, 2009c, p. 365; Wästfelt et al., 2006), patients' contribution to research activities becomes of paramount importance. Most of the sample organisations listed different fundraising activities aimed at funding research in the form of sponsorships for research projects, research programmes or clinical trials or of research career development awards. With reference to rare disease organisations, Huyard (2009a, pp. 988–989) defines "radical" those organisations—usually coordinated by one stakeholder—that have managed to secure financial resources to pursue a single goal: to support research intended to either improve treatment protocols or find a cure. What was perhaps the most interesting contribution to scientific advancement found in these organisations' narratives centred on their effort to build "boundary movements" (Brown et al., 2004; McCormick et al., 2003), that is, to build working collaborations involving patients, their families and health professionals. This seemed to happen via specifically facilitating dynamics of boundary information sharing, reported by 29 out of the 30 sample organisations:

> During November we hosted the International Neurological Conference in Stansted—sharing our 2020 Vision with the world's foremost ataxia researchers. All the scientists attending are 100% committed to researching treatments and cures for the ataxias.
>
> (Ataxia UK, 2016)

The excerpts presented above are representative of the two most common ways used by the sample organisations to frame boundary informational sharing dynamics, where patients are either addressees of scientific information or producers of experiential data of value for general practitioners, other patients and research scientists. This aligns with Rabeharisoa's (2006) interpretation of patient organisations as mediators in multi-layered interactive processes involving patients, patients' relatives, physicians and sometimes policymakers. The fact that accounts of boundary information sharing dynamics are common across rare disease organisations—and hence rare disease communities—seems to confirm that this form of involvement in scientific production constitutes an identifying element for these organisations. With reference to the mobilisation for neuromuscular diseases in France, Rabeharisoa advances that: "Patients and their families also collaborate with specialists in the production of knowledge to further their understanding of their diseases and to explore therapeutic possibilities and different ways of caring for patients" (2003,

p. 2127). In the same study, Rabeharisoa suggests that the relationship between patient organisations and health professionals has followed a trajectory where the former have progressively moved from an auxiliary position to a partnership one, with patients' knowledge increasingly affecting the advancement of biomedical research (Rabeharisoa, 2003).

In sum, in delivering their "what we have done" narrative, rare disease organisations are very likely to draw upon two core elements: a) their role as service providers for a rare disease community, with the service being provided often translating in information and b) their role as facilitators in boundary information sharing dynamics involving patients, their relatives and health professionals.

Raising Awareness in the General Public: Increasing "Disease Awareness"

In the case of rare disease organisations, a primary goal is often not so much that of reframing public perceptions but rather of being publicly acknowledged in the first place. Huyard, for instance, defines a set of rare disease organisations as "recognition claiming", with their main goal being that of "insisting that they and the disease that they represent exist and deserve attention" (2009a, p. 987). In fact, slightly more than one third of the organisations in our study directly mentioned their efforts to raise public awareness about the rare disease community they represented. Narratives here centred on the different strategies used to attract audiences and engage the general public. These strategies ranged from organising awareness days, weeks, or months to having a solid news presence, publishing popular YouTube videos, or having public awareness billboards exposed. The general effort here was that of "increasing disease awareness" (Pulmonary Fibrosis Foundation) and hence contrasting what Rabeharisoa et al. (2014b) define as the mainstream "politics of numbers" that does not help the dissemination of knowledge on individual rare diseases.

Impacting Policymaking: Increasing Awareness Among Policymakers

The very first emergence of rare disease organisations between the 1980s and the 1990s was linked to their achievements at the regulatory level when the US Orphan Drug Act first, and the EU Regulation on Orphan Medicinal Product later, facilitated the implementation of market-driven research relevant to rare diseases. In their discussion of patients' empowerment, Aymé et al. (2008, p. 2050) state that rare disease organisations

> are among the most empowered groups in the health sector, mainly as a result of their own fight for recognition and improved care. They have led the way for a new era by bridging the gap between public research, which overlooked their demands and expectations, and market-driven research, which confines research projects to those profitable enough to justify private investments.

As a matter of fact, impacting policy making has been one of the first priorities for many rare disease organisations. 11 out of the 18 organisations in the study that explicitly provided narratives of attempted or successful impact on policy making, reported raising awareness among politicians:

> Working with Parliament: In Whitehall, we work with MPs and Peers from all political parties to raise awareness of childhood cancers and of our specific campaigning issues. We also work with elected representatives in the devolved administrations.
>
> (Children with Cancer UK, 2016)

> In 2012, as a continuing public awareness program of Lynch Syndrome International the effort was expanded with 35 Governors acknowledging Lynch Syndrome Hereditary Cancer Public Awareness Day in their individual states.
>
> (Lynch Syndrome International, 2016)

Action in this area was also often framed in terms of achievements in impacting policy on public funding, to increase or save public investment relevant to a patient community. Other mentioned activities aimed at improving screening programmes, directly contributing to policy, monitoring policymaking and working at decreasing bureaucracy around clinical trials. Overall, impact on policy making was framed as aiming at "direct benefits" (e.g., financial support) and "distributive changes" (e.g., getting financial support for specific disease populations that may not have got that support in the past) (Best, 2012), and pictured policymakers as direct interlocutors.

A Typology of Rare Disease Patient Organisations

Evidence shows that providing services for patients and families and working towards enhancing scientific knowledge and clinical research are areas of action relevant across rare disease communities and organisations, with information being at the very core of both areas. On one hand, patients' and families' material and informational needs are both a key factor in the organisations' reason to be and a primary motivational element for their activist action. On the other hand, in the organisations' narratives, not only is scientific advancement supported by the organisations' fundraising activities, it is also primarily achieved by facilitating interactions between patients, families and health professionals in boundary processes of health information sharing. Patients' experiential knowledge is then deemed essential to contribute not only to diagnostic disclosure (Huyard, 2009c), but also to clinical research and treatment development (Caron-Flinterman, 2005; Panofsky, 2011).

Overall, the online public identity of rare disease organisations seems to vary primarily based on their use—or non-use—of narratives centred on raising

Table 5.4 A typology of rare disease patients' advocacy organisations.

	1. Community-oriented	*2. Policy-oriented*	*3. Public opinion-oriented*	*4. Multifunctional*
Areas of action	*Providing services* *Enhancing research*	*Providing services* *Enhancing research* *Policymaking*	*Providing services* *Enhancing research* *Public opinion*	*Providing services* *Enhancing research* *Policymaking* *Public opinion*
Organisations	Addison Disease Self Help Amyloidosis F. CLL Support Ass. National CML Society National Gaucher F. Pituary Society Short Bowel Syndrome F.	Children with Cancer UK Cystic Fibrosis Canada Cystic Fibrosis F. Fara Gaucher Ass. International Myeloma F. Leukemia & Lymphoma Lymphoma Research F. MPN Research F. Nomid Alliance	Ataxia UK HAE UK Leukaemia F. Stop CAID now Tuberous Sclerosis A.	C. Pulmonary Fibrosis Cystic Fibrosis Trust Lynch Syndrome Int. Multiple Myeloma RF Myeloma UK Pulmonary Fibrosis F. Tuberous Sclerosis A. US HAEA
Relationship organisation/ patients and family	Patients and families' material and information needs are central to reason to be and advocacy action	Patients and families' material and information needs are central to reason to be and advocacy action	Patients and families' material and information needs are central to reason to be and advocacy action	Patients and families' material and information needs are central to reason to be and advocacy action
Relationship organisation/ health professionals	Boundary information sharing dynamics are conducive to scientific advancement	Boundary information sharing dynamics are conducive to scientific advancement	Boundary information sharing dynamics are conducive to scientific advancement	Boundary information sharing dynamics are conducive to scientific advancement
Relationship organisation / policymakers	Not central	Policymakers are important addressees to achieve direct and redistributive benefits	Not central	Policymakers are important addressees to achieve direct and redistributive benefits
Relationship organisation/ general public	Not central	Not central	Increasing disease awareness in the general public is an important objective	Increasing disease awareness in the general public is an important objective

public awareness and impacting policymaking. Table 5.4 provides a typology of this identity building. Organisations that focus exclusively on providing services for patients and families and working towards enhancing scientific knowledge and clinical research can be defined as primarily "community-oriented", meaning that their identity is entirely framed around the provision of support internal to their patient community.

Organisations primarily focused on campaigning to affect the public opinion and shed light on their patient communities may be defined as "public opinion-oriented". To these organisations, increasing disease awareness in the general public is an important identity framing element that cannot be detached from their role as service providers and contributors to scientific research. Other organisations, which we can call "policy-oriented", put policy at the centre of their advocacy action. In particular, evidence shows that policymakers are often considered as central addressees to achieve "direct" and "redistributive benefits" (Best, 2012) to improve the life of rare disease patient communities. Finally, other organisations cover all areas of action, providing evidence of the fact that rare disease organisations may be "multi-directional", that is, they may be active on all different fronts of health advocacy action and directly interact with all the relevant stakeholders. These differences in identity and action give us a sense of the variety of work done by rare disease organisations—a variety that is most likely at least partially dependent on the history, visibility, diagnostics and treatment of the specific rare disease whose community they each represent.

While drawing upon research on the same sample organisations explored in the present and previous sections, the remainder of the chapter will shift the focus from identitarian narratives to technological affordances. It will draw attention to the way advocacy organisation websites provide means to engage with "connective" and "collective action" (Bennett & Segerberg, 2013; see chapter 2) centred on the diseases—and the patient communities—they represent.

Digital Mechanisms for Patient Advocacy

Health Knowledge Co-Production and Individualised Routes of Public Engagement

In our (2016) study, Cappai and I were specifically interested in the way rare disease patient organisations might exploit digital mechanisms to enhance the co-production of health knowledge involving professional experts and rare disease patients and carers, generate wider public engagement with rare disease information and advocacy, and endorse specific sources of health information relevant to rare diseases (for detailed information about the methodology we used in our research, please see Vicari & Cappai, 2016).

Our findings showed that rare disease patient organisations use a wide range of online elements to inform and engage different publics. Ready-made informative elements are the most traditional items, turning websites into repositories of data. The diagnostic information provided by organisation websites may range from descriptions of symptoms to information on inheritance patterns and disease causes, details on patients' life expectancy, patients' testimonies on symptoms, lists of relevant scientific publications, information on diagnostic centres, expert answers and FAQ sections. Treatment is usually covered with information on existing cures, general data on clinical trials, patients' testimonies on treatments and clinical trials, lists of scientific publications, expert answers, and information on support centres. Overall, these elements provide contextual information that could be of use and support for patients, patients' relatives, lay people, and general practitioners willing to know more on a specific rare disease. Details on the presence of a patients' registry are also often a key piece of information, especially to know whether a patients' database is available for future clinical trials. These pieces of information, primarily used to ground the most relevant data available on a disease, are often coupled with more dynamic elements like organisational devices (e.g., calendars and news sections), where the organisation presented future activities, video material on YouTube, Vimeo and social media feeds (e.g., RSS, Facebook, Twitter). Overall, this first set of digital mechanisms does not offer more than one-way information channels, where users are given the opportunity to browse more or less basic information and, as such, offered the possibility to engage in knowledge acquisition. Hence, these elements belong to the pool of digital mechanisms where "information can be observed moving in largely *one-way* flows from an organisation to its publics (e.g., via newsletters, closed calendars)" (Bennett & Segerberg, 2013, p. 137).

A second set of digital mechanisms is that of items that allow users to access further one-way information channels. In Cappai's and my study, two mechanisms of this type emerged as relevant in several websites: newsletter registration and email update registration. These items add an action element as they require users to take minimal action to access further information and, in so doing, they build a loose tie between the organisation and its website users. The third set of digital mechanisms that we identified in the sample websites is that of items that allow users to contact the organisation and start an information exchange. These build a collaborative channel between the end user and the organisation as they enhance communication processes that "can emerge through *interactive* information sharing" (Bennett & Segerberg, 2013, p. 137). Interactions may develop via Contact us or Registration/Log In forms or via a more or less direct involvement with the organisation's activity, like via money donations or merchandise purchases meant to contribute to fundraising. In these cases, website users, if taking the action, share more of their personal sphere with the organisation and engage in an exchange of information with it.

While the first three sets of digital mechanisms enhance one-way or two-way communication processes, the very last set enables crowdsourced communication processes. Here, users can engage with a website's internal

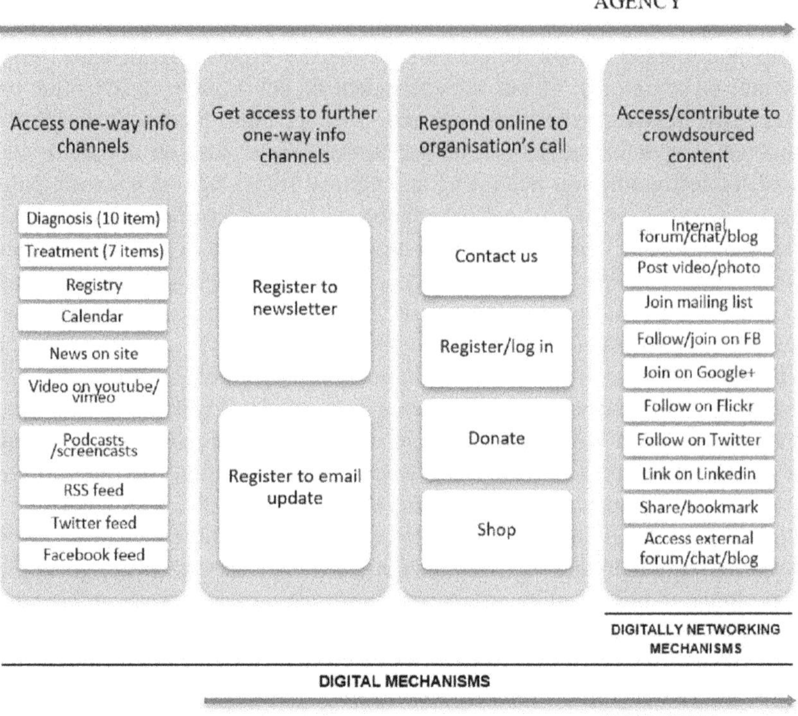

Figure 5.1 Digital Mechanisms on the websites of rare disease patient organisations.

forums, chats or blogs or share material like videos or photos. But they can also follow links to external social media platforms like the organisation's Facebook page or join its Facebook group, join the organisation's circle on Google+, follow the organisation on Flickr or Twitter, link to the organisation's LinkedIn page, join mailing lists, share or bookmark the organisation's website address or access forums, chats or blogs. These action opportunities are highly unstructured, that is, the organisation may gradually move to the background of the communication process, with different individuals and publics connecting and engaging in health personal knowledge sharing and co-production.

We can interpret these four different models of health knowledge transition (i.e., one-way communication processes) or exchange (two-way or crowdsourced communication processes) by looking at the form of engagement they require. To assess how these dynamics translate into engagement, we can draw upon two of Dahlgren's (2015) parameters of engagement: "intensity" and "depth". The former measures the degree of agency exerted by an individual to engage with an issue and the public forming around it, namely the extent to which they are free and capable to choose and contribute to debates and actions related to it.

Looked at through the intensity prism, the public engagement facilitated by digital mechanisms varies from one where individuals exert very limited agency and only engage in increasing their personal health knowledge to one where different publics potentially get involved in active discussions on health, exchanging their experiential knowledge (see Agency arrow in Table 5.1).

Evaluating the depth of engagement means measuring "how much of the self is involved" (Dahlgren, 2015), that is how much an individual exposes themselves in the act of engagement. As shown in Figure 5.1, starting from the second set of the digital mechanisms described above, website users are required to partially *become public* and share some of their personal information, with the organisation in the second and third sets of digital mechanisms, and with different publics in digitally networking mechanisms (see Publicity arrow in Figure 5.1).

In sum, the digital mechanisms used in the rare disease patient organisation websites included in our study provide evidence of at least four different types of communication processes where bottom-up selected and/or generated health knowledge is delivered to the end user, exchanged between the patient organisation and end user or crowdsourced by different end users and possibly—but not necessarily—by the patient organisation. These different channels for health knowledge transition and exchange generate different dimensions of public engagement where intensity and depth—or agency and publicity—can vary considerably.

Health Information Pathways

Not only do digital mechanisms facilitate the sharing and co-production of health knowledge via offering different ways to engage with an issue and its stakeholders—by exploiting hyperlinking structures, they also generate different health information pathways. In our (2016) study, Cappai and I tracked the online sources of information recommended by our sample organisation websites. Overall, we tracked 3,971 online sources, with 410 of them being recommended by more than one sample organisation. These ranged from websites representing other patient organisations, umbrella networks of patient organisations, national health services, public and private research centres, private companies offering patients' assistance, biomedical sources of information, news outlets, and social media platforms of different types. This indicates that rare disease patient organisations do not so much use online linking to create coalitions of patient organisations, or solidarity networks (Rogers, 2004), around patient communities but rather to redirect end users to a wide range of social actors and information sources.

Sources receiving links from more than one of the sample websites can be considered as likely influential in the overall network of rare disease patient organisations as they stand out as relevant across rare disease patient communities. Table 5.5 lists the websites that received links from six or more of our study's sample organisation websites.

Table 5.5 Top linked to websites.

Label	*Site Type*	*N Links*
facebook.com	Social Medium (social networking platform)	23
youtube.com	Social Medium (user-generated content platform)	20
clinicaltrials.gov	World registry of clinical studies	19
ncbi.nlm.nih.gov	Repository of biomedical and genomic information	17
twitter.com	Social Medium (microblogging platform)	17
fda.gov	(US) Regulatory authority for drug administration	11
cancer.gov	(US) centre for cancer research	10
nature.com	Scientific publication	10
nih.gov	(US) medical research agency	10
linkedin.com	Social Medium (professional social networking platform)	9
nlm.nih.gov	(US) library of medicine	9
rarediseases.org	(US) Umbrella network of rare disease patient organisations	9
onlinelibrary.wiley.com	Online library	8
en.wikipedia.org	Collaborative online encyclopaedia	7
geneticalliance.org	World umbrella network of rare disease patient organisations	7
justgiving.com	Social Medium (fundraising platform)	7
uk.virginmoneygiving.com	Social Medium (fundraising platform)	7
caringbridge.org	(US) Charity for patients' support	6
cdc.gov	(US) Center for disease control and prevention	6
inspire.com	Social medium (digital health platform)	6
lls.org	World health organisation	6
mayoclinic.com	(US) Medical care and Research Center	6
medicare.gov	(US) National health insurance	6
medscape.com	Scientific publication	6
nejm.org	Scientific publication	6
nhs.uk	(UK) National health service	6
nytimes.com	(US) News outlet	6
patientadvocate.org	(US) Charity for patients' support	6
patienttravel.org	(US) Charity for patients' support	6
rarediseases.info.nih.gov	(US) Center for rare disease research	6

The most evident consideration to be drawn here is that social media were more central to the network than any other online source of information or site for action. More specifically, Facebook was linked to by 23 of the sample organisations, directly followed by YouTube with 20 links, and Twitter just three positions down in the ranking with 17 links. It is certainly interesting to notice that Facebook and YouTube were sources of information slightly more likely to be linked to than institutional entities like ClinicalTrials.gov (global registry of clinical studies) and ncbi.nlm.nih.gov (repository of biomedical and genomic information) and definitely more popular than international patient organisations like raredisease.org (i.e., NORD [2021], the US Umbrella network of rare disease patient organisations). This suggests that it might be more common for rare disease patient organisations to redirect end users to social media platforms, where information is shared and co-produced by different actors in individualised processes of crowdsourced communication, rather than to entities representative of traditional scientific knowledge or institutionalised advocacy.

These results suggest that online digital networking mechanisms facilitate the development of information pathways that neither develop around clusters of patient organisations nor exclusively centralise on traditional authoritative sources of biomedical information representative of scientific knowledge and medical authority. This shows that rare disease patient organisations develop online health information pathways that often privilege crowdsourced processes of knowledge production and exchange (i.e., digitally networking mechanisms in Figure 5.1) over information seeking processes targeted at traditional scientific sources and advocacy actors.

From Organisations to Individuals and Back: Crowdsourcing and Co-Producing Rare Disease Information Online

In their work on activism in media ecosystems, Bimber, Flanagin and Stohl write:

> one of the chief obstacles to human interaction is informational: the discovery of shared interests, shared desires, or common experiences and acquaintances. Technologies that help people identify and overcome these information and communication obstacles can readily facilitate the beginnings of social behaviour.
>
> (2005, p. 382)

The empirical work presented in the last two sections focused exactly on the ways digital communication may help formal rare disease advocacy overcome informational obstacles among patients and between patients and other actors, facilitate the emergence and dissemination of patient-generated health knowledge, and provide the informational and eventually cultural context for bottom-up agency around health issues.

The digital mechanisms used in rare disease patient organisation websites generate different dynamics for health knowledge sharing (one-way communication processes), exchange (two-way communication processes) and co-production (crowdsourced communication processes), where individuals could engage in different forms of participatory practices. In fact, digital mechanisms blur the traditional boundary between private and public domains and allow the development of forms of engagement that are less personally bonding than those in traditional practices of *public* engagement. Even in the most public form of engagement—that facilitated by digitally networking mechanisms—the website end user can form loose ties both with the organisation and with other end users. By allowing greater individual control over how to engage with a health issue, this form of digital communication enhances the emergence of individualised processes that can be more inclusive than traditional forms of health advocacy. It also fundamentally increases the potential for personal networks to play a central role in health advocacy. These dynamics can be labelled as of *intraconnectivity* as they help bonding dynamics (Putnam, 2000), namely, they facilitate the emergence, development and consolidation of the illness identity (Brown & Zavestoski, 2004) of a patient community.

Seen from the lens of participatory practices, this implies that not only does digital communication in general, and digitally networking mechanisms in particular, enhance online health information seeking processes (Balka et al., 2010) and the provision and use of health information (Mager, 2009)—it also offers the context for patient organisations to form loosely networked publics that produce crowdsourced health knowledge via "second-order commonality" processes (Bimber et al., 2005, p. 372). In other words, individuals—by, for instance, participating in Facebook group discussions or Twitter hashtagged streams—can contribute to health knowledge repositories "with only partial knowledge of other participants or contributors and without a clear intention or knowledge of contributing to communal information with public goods properties" (Bimber et al., 2005, p. 372). Personal narratives of illness can then find each other online and, while certainly providing social support (Eysenbach et al., 2004) to the members of a specific patient community, they can also add elements to health knowledge relevant to that community and to the wider public.

Not only does digital networking facilitate interactions between individuals and patient organisations and among individuals; it also enacts the development of health information pathways specifically endorsed by patient organisations. The hyperlinking dynamics discussed in the last section redirected end users towards a heterogeneous range of informational sources, from the websites of other patient organisations, to those of public health institutions, private companies, scientific journals and media outlets. Within this range of actors, umbrella patient organisations were not extremely popular. This means that hyperlinking strategies did not have "aspirational" (Rogers, 2013, p. 45) goals, i.e. they did not reproduce hierarchical structures and did not represent a desire of affiliation with established, institutionalised actors. In fact, pages, groups, or discussion threads on social media platforms were often more linked to than traditional scientific resources. On one hand, end users were most likely to be redirected to crowdsourced platforms of communication where the level of moderation by the patient organisation could highly vary. In fact, the organisation's institutional presence could be totally backgrounded to free space for decentralised interactions among end users. This suggests the possibility of a fluid coexistence of "organisationally enabled" and "crowd-enabled" (Bennett & Segerberg, 2013) connective action, with individuals moving from one form of action to the other (and possibly vice versa). This also suggests that a strategic participation of health professionals and health care providers—but also regulators and policymakers[1]—in digitally networking processes (e.g., on social media platforms) would probably further help crowdsourced processes of health knowledge production, especially in the case of controversial or unresolved health issues (e.g., rare diseases).

On the other hand, links to traditional scientific resources allowed the emergence of "boundary" (Brown & Zavestoski, 2004) informational nodes that facilitated *interconnectivity*, that is, connectivity across patient communities. Most rare disease patient organisations, for instance, advocate for genetic testing and drug development, hence data on genomic information (e.g., ncbi.nlm.nih.gov) and clinical trials (e.g., clinicaltrials.gov) are central across rare disease patient communities. Hence, hyperlinking dynamics can facilitate the emergence of informational nodes that are boundary—they work as "objects that overlap different social worlds and are malleable enough to be used by different parties" (Brown & Zavestoski, 2004, p. 63), e.g., different patient groups, the biomedical community, the pharmaceutical industry and health policymakers. In this sense, hyperlinking dynamics play a strong bridging potential (Putnam, 2000).

In sum, the work presented in the last few sections seems to suggest that digital media are shaping rare disease patient advocacy in "organisationally-enabled networks", where "constituent organisations adopt the signature mode of personalizing the engagement of publics. In particular, this means deploying discourses and interactive media that offer greater choice over how people may engage" (Bennett & Segerberg, 2013, p. 48). Digital mechanisms are helping rare disease patient organisations expand discursive space, create different dimensions of public engagement and generate informational pathways where patients' experiential knowledge and scientific information are equally valued. In particular, by favouring processes of crowdsourced knowledge production and exchange, digitally networking mechanisms (e.g., Facebook pages or groups, Google+ circles, Twitter accounts or Twitter hashtagged streams) can enhance the emergence of personal narratives of illness that become central to generate and strengthen ties within a patient community, produce, share and disseminate patient-generated health epistemic knowledge and shape the context for patients' health political action.

Conclusion

This chapter has specifically focused on rare disease patient organisations to start addressing the question of how contemporary digital media may contribute to the emergence of new—or the development of pre-existing—forms of participatory cultures of health and illness. The early sections focused on the content of rare disease patient organisation websites to understand how these organisations exploit formal or institutionalised digital domains to frame their advocacy and areas of action. We saw that rare disease patient organisations tend to present themselves as providing services for patients and families and working towards enhancing scientific knowledge and clinical research. While for community-oriented organisations these are the key and only areas of actions, policy-oriented ones also focus on influencing policy making; public-oriented ones devote themselves to raising awareness in the general public and multifunctional ones are active on all fronts: community, policymaking and public awareness.

The second part of the chapter specifically explored the role of digital media in expanding health discourse practices in a way to transform traditional structures of agency in public health via the development of (1) bottom-up sharing and co-production of health knowledge, (2) health public engagement dynamics and (3) health information pathways. The work discussed here shows that digital media affordances for patient organisations go beyond the provision of social support for patient communities; they facilitate one-way, two-way and crowd-sourced processes of health knowledge sharing, exchange and co-production, provide personalised routes to health public engagement and bolster the emergence of varied pathways to health information where experiential knowledge and medical authority are often equally valued. Seen from the lens of contemporary digital activism research, these forms of organisationally-enabled connective action can help the surfacing of personal narratives that strengthen patient communities, the bottom-up production of health knowledge relevant to wider publics and the development of an informational and eventually cultural context that enhances patients' participatory action.

In the remainder of the book we will zoom in on these dynamics by specifically focusing on what could be seen as mundane participatory practices developing on contemporary digital platforms. The next chapter will begin this final part of the book's journey by specifically focusing on health-centred discursive practices on Western mainstream social media.

Note

1. EMA and FDA have been enhancing the direct involvement of patients in their activities—for example, inviting patient representatives to participate as panellists in public meetings on drug evaluation—for a few years now (Terry & Patrick-Lake, 2015). The question here is then on how such collaborations could be further enhanced via digital networking mechanisms.

Reference List

Allsop, J., Jones, K., & Baggott, R. (2004). Health consumer groups in the UK: A new social movement? *Sociology of Health and Illness*, *26*(6), 737–756.

Ataxia UK. (2016). https://www.ataxia.org.uk/

Aymé, S., Kole, A., & Graft, S. (2008). Empowerment of patients: Lessons from the rare diseases community. *Lancet*, *371*, 2048–2051.

Baggott, R., & Forster, R. (2008). Health consumer and patients' organisations in Europe: Towards a comparative analysis. *Health Expectations*, *11*, 85–94.

Balka, E., Krueger, G., Holmes, B. J., & Stephen, J. E. (2010). Situating internet use: Information-seeking among young women with breast cancer. *Journal of Computer-Mediated Communication*, *15*, 389–411.

Bennett, W. L., & Segerberg, A. (2013). *The logic of connective action: Digital media and the personalization of contentious politics*. Cambridge University Press.

Best, R. K. (2012). Disease politics and medical research funding: Three ways advocacy shapes policy. *American Sociological Review*, *77*(5), 780–803.

Bimber, B., Flanagin, A., & Stohl, C. (2005). Reconceptualizing collective action in the contemporary media environment. *Communication Theory*, *15*, 389–413.

Brown, P., & Zavestoski, S. (2004). Social movements in health: An introduction. *Sociology of Health & Illness*, *26*(6), 679–694.

Brown, P., Zavestoski, S., McCormick, S., Mayer, B., Morello-Frosch, R., & Gasior Altman, R. (2004). Embodied health movements: New approaches to social movements in health. *Sociology of Health & Illness*, *26*(12), 50–80.

Bury, M. (1982). Chronic illness as biographical disruption. *Sociology of Health & Illness*, *4*(2), 167–182.

Caron-Flinterman, J. F., Broerse, J. E. W., & Bunders, J. F. G. (2005). The experiential knowledge of patients: A new resource for biomedical research? *Social Science & Medicine*, *60*, 2575–2584.

Children with Cancer UK. (2016). https://www.childrenwithcancer.org.uk/

Dahlgren, P. (2015). *Political engagement: Charting rational and affective dimensions*. Paper presented at Media Engagement International Conference, 19 March, Lund.

Epstein, S. (2007). Patient groups and health movements. In Hackett, E. J., Amsterdamska, O., Lynch, M., & J. Wajcman (Eds.) *Handbook of science and technology studies* (3rd ed., pp. 499–539). MIT Press.

Eysenbach, G., Powell, J., Englesakis, M., Rizo, C., & Stern, A. (2004). Health related virtual communities and electronic support groups: Systematic review of the effects of online peer to peer interactions. *BMJ*, *328*, 1166.

FARA. (2016). https://www.faracharity.org/

Fox, S. (2011). Peer-to-peer healthcare: Many people: Especially those living with chronic or rare diseases: Use online connections to supplement professional medical advice. *Pew Internet & American Life Project*. www.pewinternet.org/files/oldmedia// Files/Reports/2011/Pew_P2PHealthcare_2011.pdf

Huyard, C. (2009a). Who rules rare disease associations? A framework to understand their action. *Sociology of Health & Illness*, *31*(7), 979–993.

Huyard, C. (2009b). How did uncommon disorders become "rare diseases"? History of a boundary object. *Sociology of Health & Illness*, *31*(4), 463–477.

Huyard, C. (2009c). What, if anything, is specific about having a rare disorder? Patients judgements on being ill and being rare. *Health Expectations*, *12*, 361–370.

Landzelius, K. (2006). Introduction: Patient organisation movements and new metamorphoses in patienthood. *Social Science & Medicine*, *62*, 529–537.

Lynch Syndrome International. (2016). https://lynchcancers.com/

Mager, A. (2009). Mediated health: Sociotechnical practices of providing and using online health information. *New Media and Society*, *11*(7), 1123–1142.

McCormick, S., Brown, P., & Zavestoski, S. (2003). The personal is scientific, the scientific is political: The public paradigm of the environmental breast cancer movement. *Sociological Forum*, *18*(4), 545–576.

NORD (National Organization for Rare Disorders). (2021). www.rarediseases.org

Panofsky, A. (2011). Generating sociability to drive science: Patient advocacy organizations and genetics research. *Social Studies of Science*, *41*(1), 31–57.

Papacharissi, Z. (2015). *Affective publics: Sentiment, technology, and politics*. Oxford University Press.

Petersen, A., Schermuly, A. C., & Anderson, A. (2019). The shifting politics of patient activism: From bio-sociality to bio-digital citizenship. *Health*, *23*(4), 478–494.

Putnam, R. D. (2000). *Bowling Alone*. Free Press.

Rabeharisoa, V. (2003). The struggle against neuromuscular diseases in France and the emergence of the "partnership model" of patient organisation. *Social Science & Medicine*, *57*, 2127–2136.

Rabeharisoa, V. (2006). From representation to mediation: The shaping of collective mobilization on muscular dystrophy in France. *Social Science & Medicine*, *62*, 564–576.

Rabeharisoa, V., Callona, M., Marques Filipeb, A., Arriscado Nunesc, J., Patersona, F., & Vergnauda, F. (2014b). From "politics of numbers" to "politics of singularisation": Patients' activism and engagement in research on rare diseases in France and Portugal. *BioSocieties*, *9*(2), 194–217.

Rabeharisoa, V., Moreira, T., & Akrich, M. (2014a). Evidence-based activism: Patients', users' and activists' groups in knowledge society. *BioSocieties*, *9*(2), 111–128.

Rabinow, P. (1992). Artificiality and enlightenment: From sociobiology to biosociality. In Crary, J. & Kwinter, S. (Eds.) *Incorporations* (pp. 234–252). Urzone.

Rogers, R. (2004). *Information politics on the web*. MIT Press.

Rogers, R. (2013). *Digital methods*. MIT Press.

Rose, N., & Novas, C. (2005). Biological citizenship. In Ong, A. & Collier, S. (Eds.) *Global assemblages: Technology, politics and ethics as anthropological problems* (pp. 439–463). Blackwell Publishing.

Terry, S. F., & Patrick-Lake, B. (2015). Hearing voices: FDA seeks advice from patients. *Science Translational Medicine*, *7*(313), 313ed12.

Vicari, S., & Cappai, F. (2016). Health activism and the logic of connective action: A case study of rare disease patient organisations. *Information, Communication & Society*, *19*(11), 1653–1671.

Wästfelt, M., Fadeel, B., & Henter, J. I. (2006). A journey of hope: Lessons learned from studies on rare diseases and orphan drugs. *Journal of Internal Medicine*, *260*, 1–10.

Part 3
Platforms

6 Participatory Cultures of Health and Illness on Mainstream Social Media

Introduction

Social media platforms thrive on multiplying ways for people to connect via seeking, producing, and sharing content. As discussed in Chapter 5, health content produced and shared on and across social media is increasingly relevant for ordinary users and invaluable for patient communities who rely on these platforms to access, share and process information that might be scarcely available offline. In that chapter, we saw that the opening of new routes for connecting around health topics via digital mechanisms has offered potential for illness to become an increasingly networked experience—one characterised by both personalised and fluid forms of engagement with different types of information and stakeholders. This turn has been described as strengthening the public emergence of "illness subcultures" (Conrad et al., 2016), namely, of active, and often discursive, communities whose members network around their experience and knowledge of health and illness.

Despite the growing importance of mainstream social media like Facebook, Instagram, YouTube and, more recently, TikTok (Song et al., 2021) as "spaces" to share information and learn about medicine, health and illness, social science investigations of these dynamics are still relatively limited (Lupton, 2017, p. 3). Existing research has predominantly drawn attention to the way these platforms offer "alternative" spaces to construct, narrate, and connect individual experiences of health and illness. Frohlich and Zmyslinski-Seelig (2016), for instance, investigate the use of a Facebook fan page by individuals who underwent ostomy surgeries, showing that the page's visual and textual affordances allowed users to share and comment on ostomates' selfies, ultimately helping them challenge internalised stigma. In their work on visual and multimodal social media platforms, Gonzalez-Polledo (2016) show how the pain narratives, or "pain worlds", expressed on Tumblr blogs by individuals with chronic health conditions constitute unprecedented forms of pain communication that are potentially more efficient than traditional ones, in both clinical and non-clinical contexts. According to this work, Tumblr's multimodal communication infrastructure also seems to enhance the emergence of a social dimension of chronic pain, where fragments of different life stories connect with one another in narrative networks of pain.

DOI: 10.4324/9780429469145-9

Overall, the emerging body of work investigating mainstream social media platforms as alternative spaces to experience and understand health and illness seems to suggest that the becoming public of illness subcultures has developed alongside three key dynamics. First, the health-focused virtual communities of the "Internet that was" (see Chapter 3) have been progressively replaced by new online networked structures of peer support among individuals with similar health conditions (Myrick et al., 2016; Tanis, 2008). These structures have developed within and across social media, for instance, in dedicated Facebook groups or Twitter chats or in more fluid Twitter or Instagram hashtag streams. Second, these new structures have offered renewed potential for the emergence of digital advocacy (Trevisan, 2016) and self-advocacy (Trevisan, 2017) projects centred on illness identities. Finally, traditional doctor-patient relationships have been further challenged by the exponential growth in the online availability of health information that can be easily produced, shared, and accessed by lay users (e.g., patients, carers) (Cohen & Raymond, 2011).

The following sections will touch upon these different dynamics by drawing on work that I conducted between 2015 and 2020 to investigate how Twitter users talk about the BRCA genetic mutations on the platform. Twitter cannot be considered as representative of the contemporary social media ecosystem or of any other mainstream social media because each platform has its own norms, cultures, and affordances. However, a focus on Twitter allows us to explore the potential emergence of health-centred participatory dynamics in contexts that are extremely different from the more dedicated and often contained digital spaces addressed in early Internet studies (e.g. user lists, patient or carer blogs or forums) and partially replicated in similarly contained spaces in contemporary social media platforms (e.g., Facebook pages of groups, Tumblr blogs).

While zooming in on Twitter content produced in relation to the BRCA mutations between 2013 and 2017, this chapter focuses on four dimensions that have been identified in the previous chapters as extremely relevant to digital participatory cultures, health advocacy or both: content curation, framing practices, storytelling and epistemic work. After providing contextual information about the BRCA gene mutations as a health condition, the next sections will first explore curation and framing practices by drawing upon a longitudinal research project that examined BRCA-focused tweets posted on the platform in 2013 and 2015 (for detailed information about the methodology used in the project, please see Vicari, 2017). The following two sections will draw attention to storytelling and epistemic dynamics by reflecting on a subsequent piece of research where I investigated BRCA tweets from 2017 (for detailed information about the methodology used in this research, please see Vicari, 2020). Finally, by bringing together the considerations drawn in relation to BRCA content curation, framing, storytelling and epistemic work, the remainder of the chapter will provide a set of reflections on how mainstream social media platforms contribute to participatory cultures of health and illness.

BRCA, Angelina Jolie and Twitter

BRCA1 and BRCA2 are hereditary genetic mutations that increase the risk to develop breast, ovarian and other types of cancer (National Cancer Institute, 2021). These mutations are diagnosed by mapping family histories of cancer and performing predictive genetic testing. "BRCA" became a topic of wider public interest when in May 2013 and March 2015 US celebrity Angelina Jolie wrote in the New York Times about being a carrier of the BRCA1 gene mutation. In 2013, Jolie would say: "I have always told them [my children] not to worry, but the truth is I carry a 'faulty' gene, BRCA1, which sharply increases my risk of developing breast cancer and ovarian cancer". In her op-eds (2013, 2015), Jolie explained her choice to undergo prophylactic surgery—a mastectomy and the removal of ovaries and fallopian tubes—to prevent cancer. Following the first op-ed, the story was picked up by news and entertainment media in both Western and Asian periodicals, with the celebrity's picture appearing on the covers of People and Time magazines and the content of her op-ed remaining of news value for months (Borzekowski et al., 2014; Evans et al., 2014; Kamenova et al., 2014; Noar et al., 2015). Jolie's story was given primarily positive offline (Kamenova et al., 2014) and online (Dean, 2016) institutional media coverage, with however little attention being drawn to the rarity of her genetic condition (Borzekowski et al., 2014). Following Jolie's first op-ed, a so-called "Angelina effect" (Kluger et al., 2013) was measurable in the steady increase in requests for genetic testing around the world (Barton, 2013; Dunlop et al., 2014; Evans et al., 2014; Kosenko et al., 2016; Mehta, 2013; Neporent, 2013) and in online information seeking about it (Noar et al., 2015).

BRCA is a very interesting case study to understand how mainstream social media platforms shape public or semi-public conversations within illness subcultures because the BRCA Twitter thread has now been active for almost a decade: it pre-existed Jolie's op-eds and continued its activity through the peaks—and the "ad-hoc publics" (Bruns & Burgess, 2011)—generated by the op-eds themselves. In other words, what we may see as a fluid and resilient networked public has been talking about BRCA on Twitter since before 2013. The BRCA condition is also extremely interesting in terms of exploring participatory cultures of health and illness because BRCA advocacy groups have been active for some time now. In 2013, for instance, some of these groups were involved in the US judicial case "Association for Molecular Pathology versus Myriad Genetics" that challenged the legitimacy of pharmaceutical company Myriad Genetics' human gene patents. Among other forms of action, BRCA activists took part in the "Human gene patent rally" on 15 April 2013, when arguments against gene patents were being presented to the Court in Washington D. C. (Carmody & Sartor, 2013).

Curation

Given its sociotechnical infrastructure, Twitter content undergoes "intense curation practices" (Bennett et al., 2014, p. 245). On one hand, the platform itself shapes content via its algorithmic recommendation systems that, for instance, highlight "What's happening", "Who to follow", and "Topics to follow" on the basis of the platformisation logic that we discussed in Chapter 2. On the other hand, users can curate content through the use of conversational markers: broadcasters increase the visibility of other users and of the content these users share on the platform by retweeting or @ mentioning them. Those who are most likely to be retweeted or mentioned turn into gatekeepers of information because the content they produce is most likely to become visible on the platform.

When I first approached BRCA content on Twitter, I specifically focused on longitudinal curation dynamics because I wanted to bring insight into the way broadcasters and gatekeepers within the BRCA Twitter public might have evolved over time. Existing research shows that the networked structure of contemporary health-centred online communities often foregrounds some users over others. As McCosker suggests: "connectors, intermediaries or influencers designate those who act with a degree of vernacular authority to bridge professional and non-professional divides, establish and sustain supportive online communities and help to frame and re-frame others' experiences of mental ill-health" (2018, p. 4751). By focusing on broadcasting and gatekeeping dynamics, I aimed to identify this authority in Twitter conversations about BRCA and track how it evolved between 2013 and 2015.

Broadcasters and Gatekeepers of BRCA Content in 2013

Table 6.1 maps[1] the top broadcasters of BRCA content between 14/04 and 13/06/2013, namely, starting one month before the publication of Jolie's first op-ed and ending one month after it. "Top broadcasters" are those users who most often used conversational markers, namely, "RT" (retweet), "@" and "via'. The "via" marker used to appear in tweets automatically generated when clicking on a web page's share button. The last three columns of Table 6.1 list the top 10 broadcasters in the month before Jolie's announcement (i.e., 14/04–13/05/2013), during the first 8 days after the piece's publication, when the daily number of tweets was higher than ever before (i.e., 14/05–21/05/2013), and in the remaining period (i.e., 22/05–13/06/2013). The table shows that different actors gained influence over time, with only US-based advocacy organisation Breast Cancer Action (i.e., BCAction) recurring before, during and after the publication of Jolie's op-ed (bolded).

It is interesting to notice that among the broadcasters that were prominent across two of the three periods (underlined), advocacy organisations (i.e., abcd, BCCampaign, BRCAUmbrella, Florida Force and Kartemquin, and Tealtoes) played a central role. These actors were extremely active in retweeting, mentioning and via-ing other users of the platform. Broadcasting amplifies certain voices among others, giving them increased visibility. Those who gain this increased visibility turn into gatekeepers because their content and their identity gains prominence in the conversational network.

Table 6.1 Top broadcasters of BRCA content in the 2013 sample period.

Rank	*Before*	*During*	*After*
1	FloridaForce	Shirakrance	AstleyClarke
2	Eperlste	darwinianfail	Yablon
3	**BCAction**	abcdiagnosis	**BCAction,** JoannaRudnick
4	Individual_6	Yablon	BRCAGeneAware
5	BRCAUmbrella	ABHuret	BRCAUmbrella
6	SLLitchy	FacingOurRisk	abcdiagnosis, PennMedicine, Pink_Hope
7	chemobrainfog	**BCAction**, PitzPoodle, Tealtoes	Individual_3
8	PinkMoonLovelie	CheckYourGenes, DrAttai, Individual_3	BRCAStudyBC, Jamesian, Kartemquin
9	individual_1, Tealtoes	chemobrainfog	retnobi91
10	BRCAinfo	BRCAinfo	DrAttai, FloridaForce, GDM80, yale79DAV

Table 6.2 Top gatekeepers of BRCA content in the 2013 sample period.

Rank	*Before*	*During*	*After*
1	BCAction	TIME	**ACLU**
2	**ACLU**	HealthRanger	myriadgenetics
3	kara_dioguardi	theRightSteph	AP
4	FacingOurRisk	**ACLU**	KitFrieden
5	myriadgenetics	causes	BCAction
6	sandrasparkly	CR_UK	LizSzabo
7	Individual_6	ClevelandClinic	FacingOurRisk
8	elizabethiorns	katiecouric	BCCampaign
9	mrgunn	DrOz	Amyverner
10	ACLULive	AstroKatie	xeni

Table 6.2 maps the evolution of the BRCA Twitter conversational network over the 2013 sample period.

But let us have a closer look at the gatekeeping dynamics specifically developing in the three different time periods.

Before

Before Jolie's public announcement, US-based advocacy organisations Breast Cancer Action and Force (i.e., FacingOurRisk) and pharmaceutical company Myriad Genetics (i.e, myriadgenetics) acted as prominent gatekeepers (underlined in Table 6.2), together with a few individual Twitter users. Myriad Genetics' gatekeeping prominence is directly linked to events happening on the ground in relation to the ongoing judicial case "Association for Molecular Pathology versus Myriad Genetics", where the ACLU itself served as counsel for the plaintiffs. As mentioned above, the case challenged the legitimacy of Myriad Genetics' human gene patents and was specifically relevant to the BRCA Twitter public as human gene patents increased the price of BRCA genetic testing, reducing its accessibility. In fact, Myriad Genetics played a prominent role as a target of tweets campaigning against human gene patenting.

During

In the conversational network developing during the first eight days after the publication of Jolie's op-ed, the ambient nature of Twitter conversational practices emerged with the coming to prominence of mainstream media outlets (i.e., Time) among advocacy organisations (i.e., CR_UK, or Cancer Research UK), individual advocates (i.e., HealthRanger) news editors (i.e., theRightSteph) and public figures (i.e., journalist Katie Couric and astrophysicist Katherine Mack, or AstroKatie). In fact, with the mediatisation of Jolie's BRCA narrative, traditional gatekeepers temporarily entered the BRCA Twitter stream, combining with—but not replacing—new ones, in a "hybrid news system" (Chadwick, 2013).

After

Over the remaining period, Myriad Genetics and ACLU became by far the most prominent gatekeepers. On 13 June 2013, the US Supreme Court decided that naturally occurring DNA sequences, like BRCA1 and BRCA2, could no longer be patented. This caused a sudden rise in Twitter activity on 13 June 2013, foregrounding ACLU and Myriad Genetics in the "After" Twitter conversational network. The advocacy organisations in leading gatekeeping roles before the publication of Jolie's op-ed (i.e., FacingOurRisk and BCAction) also re-emerged here (underlined in Table 6.2) among a number of new individual Twitter users.

Overall, through Jolie's first public announcement, health advocacy organisations were the primary curators (i.e., broadcasters and gatekeepers) of BRCA-related Twitter content. The BRCA stream was then mainly sourced via "organisationally-enabled connective action" (Bennett & Segerberg, 2013), or via connective action mobilised by "non-elite" collective actors, namely, advocacy organisations. To be clear, in this context, "non-elite" stands for entities who are not usually playing a key role in curating the production and diffusion of public content—a role that has been traditionally covered by news media outlets, prominent public figures and institutions. In line with what we discussed in Chapter 5 in relation to rare disease advocacy, these findings also suggest that in 2013 Twitter was a communication and mobilisation platform clearly embedded in the work of BRCA advocacy organisations, especially in the US context. Jolie's announcement had a short-term effect on curation dynamics: it temporarily introduced a hybrid dimension in the BRCA Twitter stream, with mainstream media sharing gatekeeping prominence with advocacy organisations and individual Twitter users.

Broadcasters and Gatekeepers of BRCA Content in 2015

Data from 2015 show that in a two-year span, curation practices within the BRCA Twitter stream changed dramatically. The last three columns of Table 6.3 list top broadcasters in the month before Jolie's second announcement (i.e., 24/02–23/03/2015), during the first four days following its publication, when the daily number of tweets was higher than ever before (i.e., 24/03–27/03/2015), and in the remaining period (i.e., 28/03–23/04/2015). Five out of the six top broadcasters who recurred before, during and after Jolie's announcement in 2015 (bolded) were individual self-declared patient advocates mobilising around BRCA conditions and hereditary cancer (i.e., BRCAresponder, karenBRCAMTL, BRCAinfo and NickiDurlester) or Lynch Syndrome[2] and hereditary cancer (i.e., ShewithLynch). Two out of the three broadcasters recurring in two periods (underlined) were also breast cancer individual advocates (i.e., LguzzardiM, Individual_5).

Conversational dynamics also varied compared to 2013. In fact, Table 6.4 shows that five individual self-declared patient advocates (i.e., karenBRCAMTL, BRCAresponder, BRCAinfo, Lguzzardi and ShewithLynch) recurred as top gatekeepers over the entire sample period.

But let us focus more specifically on the gatekeeping dynamics emerging in the three different time periods.

Table 6.3 Top broadcasters of BRCA content in the 2015 sample period.

Rank	*Before*	*During*	*After*
1	**BRCAresponder**	**BRCAresponder**	**karenBRCAMTL**
2	**BRCAUmbrella**	**BRCAUmbrella**	**BRCAresponder**
3	**ShewithLynch**	**ShewithLynch**	**ShewithLynch**
4	**karenBRCAMTL**	DoveMed	**BRCAUmbrella**
5	Individual_2	**BRCAinfo, karenBRCAMTL**	Individual_5
6	OvarianCancerUK	Pinkandbluedoc	**BRCAinfo**
7	**BRCAinfo**	Individual_5	**NickiDurlester**
8	pinkandbluedoc	Tmskr401	LguzzardiM
9	**NickiDurlester**	**NickiDurlester**	Hc_chat
10	LguzzardiM	double_whammied	Individual_4, MHBTmovie

Table 6.4 Top gatekeepers of BRCA content in the 2015 sample period.

Rank	*Before*	*During*	*After*
1	**karenBRCAMTL**	**BRCAresponder**	Facebook
2	BRCAUmbrella	mindykaling	**karenBRCAMTL**
3	**BRCAresponder**	OvarianCancerUK	**BRCAresponder**
4	OvarianCancerUK	BRCAUmbrella	**ShewithLynch**
5	**BRCAinfo**	nytimes	**LguzzardiM**
6	**LguzzardiM**	**LguzzardiM**	**BRCAinfo**
7	facebook	**BRCAinfo**	ColorGenomics
8	**ShewithLynch**	**karenBRCAMTL**	Pinkandbluedoc
9	ClairaHermet	BBC_WHYS	MyGeneCounsel
10	beBRCAware	**ShewithLynch**	EricTopol

Before

Before the exposure of Jolie's story, several individual patient advocates (e.g., karenBRCAMTL, BRCAresponder, BRCAinfo, LguzzardiM, ShewithLynch) played top gatekeeping roles along with only two advocacy organisations (i.e., BRCAUmbrella and OvarianCancerUK). Facebook was among the top mentioned sources, primarily due to a high number of tweets mentioning Facebook as part of a campaign against the removal of mastectomy photos on BRCA Facebook pages.

During

Like in 2013, with the publication of Jolie's op-ed, traditional news outlets (i.e., New York Times and BBC) temporarily reached gatekeeping prominence. They populated a highly hybrid gatekeeping system along US celebrity Mindy Kaling, advocacy organisations Ovarian Cancer UK, and the scientific journal JAMA.

After

During the remaining period, individual patient advocates (e.g., karenBRCAMTL, BRCAresponder, ShewithLynch, LguzzardiM, BRCAinfo, MyGeneCounsel) played an even stronger gatekeeping role than before the publication of Jolie's piece, with Facebook re-emerging as the target of campaigning against the removal of mastectomy photos on BRCA Facebook pages.

Overall, these dynamics show a dramatic shift in Twitter curation practices occurring between 2013 and 2015, with individual patient advocates replacing advocacy organisations as top curators—in broadcasting and gatekeeping roles—of the BRCA Twitter stream. This change in curation practices then shows that in a two-year span, connective action sourcing the BRCA Twitter stream went from being primarily "organisationally-enabled" to essentially "crowd-enabled" (Bennett & Segerberg, 2013). Both Jolie's announcements added a hybrid dimension in gatekeeping dynamics but did not inhibit the role of pre-existing curators.

We may speculate that this shift in connective action depends on both cultural and socio-technical factors. On the one hand, it is likely that a longitudinal rise in public awareness about BRCA-related topics—probably also linked to the exposure of Jolie's story—led to the progressive emergence of personalised forms of engagement with them. On the other hand, the manifestation of these personalised forms of engagement was enhanced by Twitter's sociotechnical infrastructure that allowed non-elite *individual* actors (i.e., patient advocates) to engage in content curation processes that two years earlier were controlled by non-elite *collective* actors (i.e., advocacy organisations). In other words, these findings suggest that not only can Twitter broadcast networks open up space for minorities' viewpoints (Benkler, 2006; Jackson & Foucault Welles, 2015, 2016), they can also allow significant power shifts between collective and individual actors within minorities themselves.

Frames

The curation dynamics prompted by Twitter users via broadcasting and gatekeeping lead to the emergence of dominant narratives, or frames, that work "through persistent patterns of selection, interpretation, emphasis, exclusion, and retention" (Meraz & Papacharissi, 2013, p. 143). Frames, as composite cognitive elements, develop via the use of language-specific devices like hashtags. Hashtags segment broad issue publics, like the BRCA public, around topic-specific streams. By looking at hashtag co-occurrence networks, or the combined use of different hashtags within a Twitter stream, it is then possible to map the articulation of broad issues along topical dimensions, and identify dominant narratives associated with them. Focusing on the tweets showing the curation dynamics discussed in the previous section, I explored the use of hashtags to frame BRCA as a health condition. The next two subsections discuss the different frames emerging before, during and after the publication of Jolie's op-eds in 2013 and 2015.

BRCA Frames in 2013

Table 6.5 maps the top hashtag co-occurrences in the 2013 sample period and shows that the only hashtag pair recurring over the whole period (bolded) associated the BRCA gene mutation with breast cancer.

Before

Before heightened mainstream media exposure due to Jolie's op-ed, the BRCA gene mutation was primarily discussed in terms of gene patents and their implications. The BRCA Twitter stream was almost entirely focused on

Table 6.5 Hashtag pairs with top 10 frequencies over the 2013 sample period.

Rank	*Before*		*During*		*After*	
	#1	*#2*	*#1*	*#2*	*#1*	*#2*
1	BRCA	SCOTUS	**BRCA**	**breastcancer**	BRCA	SCOTUS
2	**BRCA**	**breastcancer**	BRCA	AngelinaJolie	**BRCA**	**breastcancer**
3	BRCA	genepatent	BRCA1	cancer	BRCA	genes
4	BRCA	genepatents	BRCA1	breastcancer	SCOTUS	genes
5	BRCA	cancer	BRCA1	AngelinaJolie	SCOTUS	Myriad
6	BRCASCOTUS	Myriadbreastcancer	BRCA1	breast	BRCA	BCSM
7	BRCA	hgprally	BRCA	BCSM	BRCABCSM	genepatents breastcancer
8	SCOTUSSCOTUS	genepatentsgenepatent	BRCA	mastectomy	BRCA	Myriad
9	BRCA	previvor	BRCA	cancer	SCOTUS	breastcancer
10	SCOTUS	hgprally	breastcancer	AngelinaJolie	genepatents	DNA

Myriad Genetics' ownership of the BRCA gene patents, with attention being drawn to the ongoing legal case. #hgprally, for instance—that in the first hashtag network frequently co-occurred with the top hashtags #BRCA and #SCOTUS (i.e., Supreme Court of the United States)—was an event hashtag used during the Human gene patent rally of 15 April 2013. The rally, organised by Breast Cancer Action, took place on the steps of the U.S. Supreme Court while arguments against gene patents were being presented to the Court (Carmody and Sartor, 2013). Hashtags like #gene, #genepatents, #genepatent, and #previvor were also frequently linked to #BRCA and #SCOTUS.

During

Jolie's announcement had short term effects, the most evident of which being a sudden shift toward Jolie's BRCA-related narrative, with the foregrounding of the BRCA1 gene mutation over the BRCA2 one and of prophylactic mastectomy as a preventive measure. Finally, Jolie's story enhanced the emergence of dedicated Twitter chats (i.e., BCSM and BasserBRCA).

After

In the remaining period, top hashtag pairs reframed the BRCA issue stream around genes, gene patents and the trial involving Myriad Genetics, like in the period prior to the publication of Jolie's editorial, indicating that the Angelina effect on framing dynamics was extremely short-termed.

Hence, across the publication of Jolie's first op-ed, the BRCA Twitter stream developed around both content-based frames descriptive of real-world events on the ground and more volatile and short-lived content-based frames emerging with Jolie's story. These dynamics indicate that Twitter functioned primarily as a "news reporting mechanism" (Papacharissi & De Fatima Oliveira, 2012), hosting, for instance, the live coverage of the Human gene patent rally but also enhancing the inclusion of Jolie-related BRCA articulations. The co-presence of both framing dynamics suggests that users engaged in connective action with different levels of agency, with Twitter having both mobilising (Bennett & Segerberg, 2013) and ambient (Hermida, 2010; Bruns & Burgess, 2012) functions.

BRCA Frames in 2015

Table 6.6 lists the top hashtag pairs over the 2015 sample period. Data show that in 2015 not only was the BRCA gene mutation regularly associated with breast cancer, like in 2013; it was also constantly linked to the hashtag #BCSM, tagging a breast cancer Twitter chat (bolded).

Before

Looking at Table 6.6, it is evident that in 2015, before Jolie's announcement, the BRCA Twitter stream was mainly developing around breast cancer narratives. But while mastectomy was a popular co-occurring hashtag already in 2013, the new

Table 6.6 Hashtag pairs with top 10 frequencies over the 2015 sample period.

	Before		*During*		*After*	
	#1	*#2*	*#1*	*#2*	*#1*	*#2*
1	**BRCA**	**BCSM**	BRCA	AngelinaJolie	**BRCA**	**BCSM**
2	**BRCA**	**breastcancer**	BRCA	cancer	BCSM	breastcancer
3	BCSM	breastcancer	BRCA	ovariancancer	mastectomy	breastcancer
4	BRCA	ovariancancer	**BRCA**	**breastcancer**	**BRCA**	**breastcancer**
5	BRCA	Mastectomy	BRCA	HCChat	BCSM	mastectomy
6	mastectomy	breastcancer	BRCA	hereditarycancer	BRCA	mastectomy
7	BCSM	mastectomy	**BRCA**	**BCSM**	BRCA	facebook
8	BRCA	bckills	cancer	AngelinaJolie	mastectomy	facebook
9	BRC Ametsmonday metsmonday	Lynchsyndrome bckills dontignorestageiv	AngelinaJolie	ovariancancer	BCSM breastcancer BCSM BRCA breastcancer facebook	facebook facebook photosphotos photosphotos
10	BRCA	facebook	BRCA	HCChat		Lynchsyndrome

frequent use of the hashtag #metsmonday, tagging a Monday chat for people with metastatic cancer, with #dontignorestageiv and #bckills (see Table 6.6) signals the emergence of new framing dynamics. It indicates a turn in the discussion towards more specialist themes associated with breast cancer; themes more popular within the environmental, or political, breast cancer movement (Klawiter, 1999; McCormick, et al., 2003) than in mainstream representations of breast cancer (see Chapter 3). This specialist turn is also signalled by the frequent association of BRCA with Lynch Syndrome, as this association indicates awareness of similarities between the BRCA gene mutations and other genetic mutations increasing cancer risk (e.g., Lynch Syndrome). These findings suggest the appropriation of the BRCA Twitter stream by activist actors and a consequent shift towards the emergence of activist action frames. In fact, these framing dynamics suggest that by 2015, the BRCA Twitter stream had expanded its scope as an awareness system, hosting more dynamic articulations of BRCA-related topics than in 2013.

During

In the short term, Jolie's announcement, like in 2013, mainly introduced frame articulations directly linked to Jolie's BRCA narrative. First, it drew attention to the hereditary nature of the BRCA gene mutation via the use of #BRCA with #HCChat, a Twitter chat focused on hereditary cancer, and #hereditarycancer. Second, it foregrounded inspirational hashtags like #knowledgeispower. Third, it drew attention to ovarian cancer-related narratives via hashtags like #HBOC, tagging hereditary breast and ovarian cancer tweets, and #gyncsm, a Twitter chat for individuals talking about gynecological cancers.

After

Finally, similar dynamics to those described for the period before the publication of Jolie's op-ed are evident in the hashtag network developing towards the end of the 2015 sample period. There, #mastectomy, #breastcancer and #BCSM are frequently associated to #BRCA and Lynch syndrome is again linked to the BRCA gene mutation. In this hashtag network, #facebook also gains visibility due to the ongoing campaign against Facebook's removal of mastectomy photos described in the analysis of curation dynamics.

Overall, these framing dynamics suggest that while in April-June 2013 the BRCA Twitter stream primarily functioned as a news reporting mechanism centred around content-based frames, in February-April 2015 it worked more as an "awareness system" (Hermida, 2010) where narratives developed around specialist topical dimensions. In both sample periods, the exposure of Jolie's story temporarily introduced frame articulations directly linked to Jolie's BRCA narrative. These findings, coupled with previous results on shifting curation practices, picture the BRCA Twitter stream as developing, between 2013 and 2015, via the foregrounding of personalised over collective forms of engagement, with patient advocates emerging as top curators of specialist narratives of health and illness.

Storytelling

As we discussed in Chapter 3, after Bury's (1982) sociological interpretation of illness as a "biographical disruption", growing research, by both sociologists and medical professionals, has pointed to the relevance of "illness narratives" (Hydén, 1997) in coping with the challenges brought by disease. According to this comprehensive body of work, the telling of stories helps individuals come to terms with their condition, redefine their social relations and reaffirm their sense of self (Bury, 2001).

Digital storytelling has been investigated as typical of online health-focused conversations since the early 2000s, when scholars started to draw attention to the way people share stories of health, illness and caring on the Internet in general (Hardey, 2002) or on online social spaces like blogs (Orgad, 2005), or multiuser environments (Bers, 2009) in particular. As discussed in Chapter 4, in her pivotal work on online breast cancer blogs, Orgad describes storytelling as the act of creating "a framework that would capture . . . multiple and scattered events . . . An attempt to produce a self-story that helps its teller and her listeners to make sense of her experience" (2005, p. 43). Often drawing upon this pivotal work, social science research has used the storytelling paradigm to provide insight into the potential for contemporary mainstream social media to enhance the emergence of communities interacting around personal narratives of health and illness, very much in line with what Akrich (2010) has defined as "communities of experience" (see Chapter 4). This research is providing in-depth explorations of the development of non-traditional forms of storytelling, where visual content plays a key role.

Given that social media research has often defined Twitter as a "storytelling medium" (Papacharissi, 2016) or a "storytelling machine" (Rogers, 2019), I decided to assess the extent to which the BRCA Twitter public used storytelling in its content sharing practices. To do so, I focused on BRCA content shared on Twitter during one month of activity unrelated to events of news value: 30 March–29 April 2017. My analysis shows that in that period the BRCA public was actually more than twice as likely to produce content that excluded rather than included instances of storytelling (Table 6.7).

Table 6.7 Personal storytelling and communication practices in the 2017 sample period.

		Communication practice		*Grand Total*
		Original tweeting	*Automated sharing (i.e., RT or button sharing)*	
Personal storytelling	*yes*	268 (28.42%)	675 (71.58%)	*943 (100%)*
	no	636 (33.39%)	1,269 (66.61%)	*1,905 (100%)*
	Grand Total	904 (31.74%)	1,944 (68.26%)	*2,848 (100%)*

BRCA Stories of Others

Reading through the tweets that did report fragments of personal narratives, I soon realised that I was rarely coming across first-person accounts. In fact, more than 70% of these tweets were the result of automatic or semi-automatic sharing (Table 6.7), hence messages relaying someone else's story. These practices can be seen as a form of intertextuality: a text is being selected and re-presented in the same context (i.e., retweeted) or in a different one (i.e., button shared from their original webpage). The positionality of these tweets' authors, however, remains ambiguous: while enhancing the visibility of BRCA content, these authors did not invest in commenting on, expressing an opinion about or reshaping it. In other words, via these automated sharing practices, tweeters could draw attention to the BRCA subculture, without having to expose their own relationship with BRCA or, where relevant, their "self-story" (Orgad, 2005) as part of the BRCA subculture itself.

When authors visibly engaged with the stories they tweeted (i.e., via original messages), they used different forms of intertextuality to position themselves in relation to the content they shared. User 3 (Figure 6.1),[3] for instance, a seemingly ordinary user, expressed intimacy with the subject at the centre of the story they shared by addressing them as "a friend of mine". Similarly, non-profit organisation Hereditary Cancer (Figure 6.2) expressed sympathy for US media celebrity Lesley Murphy "for her public display of bravery", namely, for narrating her BRCA self-story on her Instagram account (and other media outlets). Hereditary Cancer (Figure 6.3) visualised this closeness with the "two hearts" emoji, here working as a "marker of emotion" (Bellander & Landqvist, 2020), a device used to emphasise affect. Hereditary Cancer, however, like the collective account Genomic Alliance, also relied on this storytelling to raise awareness on a BRCA-related issues (e.g., cancer preventative surgery in Figure 6.2, male breast cancer in Figure 6.3).

This use of third person storytelling resonates with Trevisan's (2017, p. 191) findings on the ever growing "advocacy technique of . . . crowd-sourcing, organizing, and disseminating personal life stories online".

User 3
@Partici58626867
This is a nice piece written by a friend of mine, on facing challenges and confidently fighting back.
medium.com/@sazcoster/ble ...

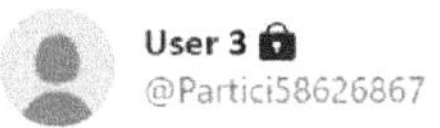

Figure 6.1 Storytelling tweet (1) (anonymised and paraphrased).

Source: (URL to Koster, 2017).

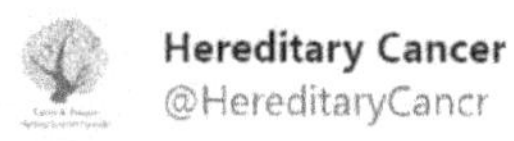

Hereditary Cancer
@HereditaryCancr
Shout out to @LesleyMurph for her public display of bravery following her prophylactic, bilateral mastectomy #BRCA #previvor
Lesley Murphy @LesleyMurph · Apr 17, 2017
My Sunday best, or what I could manage to put on today with limited arm movements. My mom washed and dried my ... ift.tt/2oCbPym
7:06 PM · Apr 17, 2017 · Twitter for iPhone

Figure 6.2 Storytelling tweet (2).

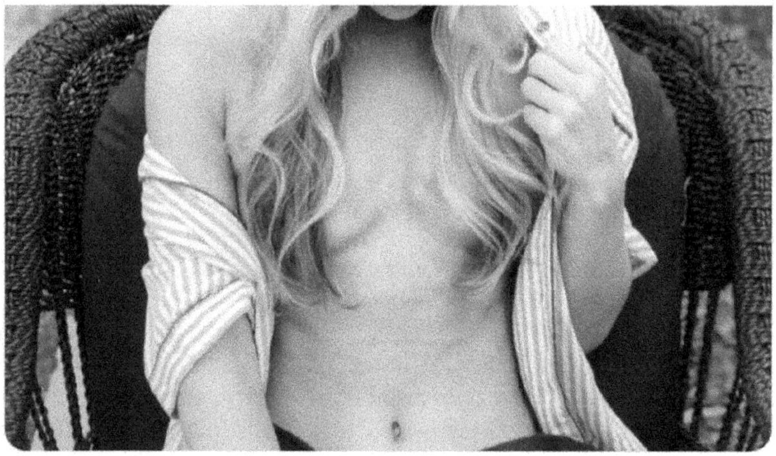

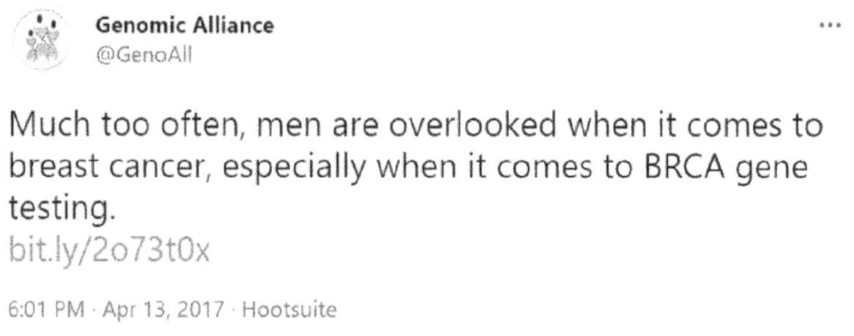

Genomic Alliance
@GenoAll
Much too often, men are overlooked when it comes to breast cancer, especially when it comes to BRCA gene testing.
bit.ly/2o73t0x
6:01 PM · Apr 13, 2017 · Hootsuite

Figure 6.3 Storytelling tweet (3).

Source: (URL to Tucker, 2016).

First-Person BRCA Stories

Given that less than one third of the storytelling tweets in the study were original messages (see Table 6.7), first person accounts were obviously not common. However, among these, I could identify iconic instances of storytelling, where fragments of life events were related together to draw a story along a temporal continuum (Orgad, 2005). User 4, for instance, microblogged her BRCA self-story and used it with the "heart" emoji, again a marker of emotion, to express sympathy to User 10 (Figure 6.4).

Traditional storytelling seemed, however, to evolve in a variety of ways. Sometimes it emerged as part of "influencer" work. Lesley Murphy (Figure 6.5)

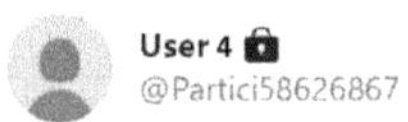

@User10 I am a survivor My mum and sister passed from it I am BRCA1 Glad you are fine

2:55 PM · Jun 23, 2021 · Twitter Web App

Figure 6.4 Storytelling tweet (4) (anonymised and paraphrased).

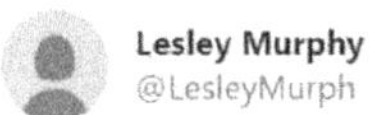

My 1st post about my surgery is up! Raw thoughts, feelings and new photos on the blog! Photo by @uamshealth bit.ly/brca-2-mastect... #bcra

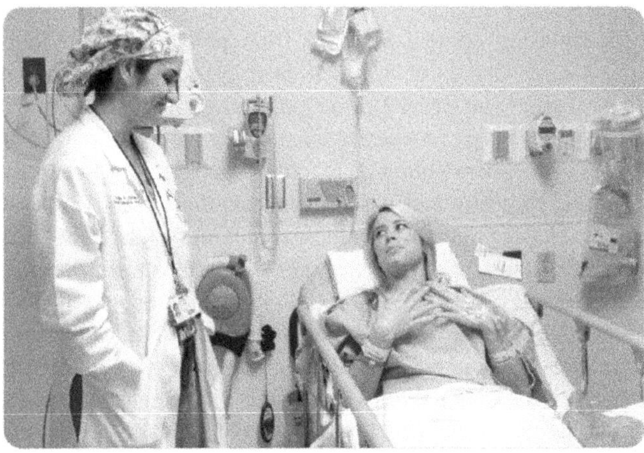

7:04 PM · Apr 21, 2017 · Twitter Web Client

Figure 6.5 Storytelling tweet (5).

Source: (URL to Murphy, 2017).

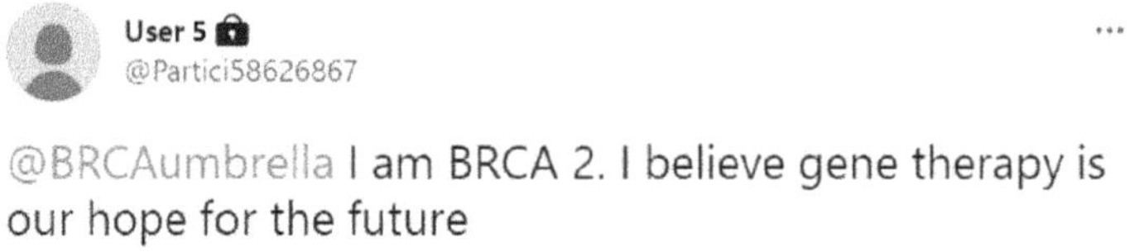

@BRCAumbrella I am BRCA 2. I believe gene therapy is our hope for the future

Figure 6.6 Storytelling tweet (6) (anonymised and paraphrased).

live streamed her BRCA self-story, reshaping her "coherent branded identity" (McCosker, 2018, p. 4752) around it. Intertextuality here allowed Murphy to mention @uamshealth, (i.e., the University of Arkansas for Medical Sciences, where the surgery supposedly took place) and to hop with her readers on to her Instagram account for the live streaming of her BRCA self-story

In some cases, first person storytelling manifested itself in subtler formats. In the tweet presented in Figure 6.6, for instance, "I am BRCA 2" translates into a series of unsaid events, namely, "I experienced cancer (directly or via a member of my family), I did a genetic test, I found out I have the BRCA 2 gene mutation". The accent here is however not so much on those scattered events, their sequence or the actors who participated in them; it is on what follows in the tweet: "I believe gene therapy is our hope for the future". Storytelling is then here functional to frame the author's identity and "lay expertise" (Hardey, 2002); in this tweet, User 5 was saying: "I am x, hence I am entitled to say y".

BRCA Non-Stories

Most tweets reporting content different from personal storytelling directly drew upon external sources of information (e.g., conference presentation in Tweet 1, journal article in Tweet 2), with authors again usually (i.e., 67% of the times, see Table 6.7) either retweeting existing content (Figure 6.7) or sharing URLs via the Twitter share button on external webpages (Figures 6.8 and 6.9).

It is interesting to notice that while relying on these platform-automated or semi-automated sharing dynamics, authors sometimes engaged in active textual crafting by, for instance, inserting hashtags (#BreastCancer, #ProstateCancer, #BRCA and #Genetics in the tweet shown in Figure 6.8 but not in the automatically generated text shown in Figure 6.9) or deleting bits of the original text (e.g., "—PubMed—NCBI" in Figure 6.9 but not in the tweet in Figure 6.8).

In entering or navigating the Twittersphere via these automated or semi-automated sharing practices, non-storytelling content was often simply synthetized and translated in a way to comply with—and make the most of—platform norms. In this transition, traditional "markers of direct reference" (Bellander & Landqvist, 2020, p. 5)—that is, linguistic devices that indicate the sources of the information being shared—are replaced by what we may define as "platform markers of reference", e.g., shortened URLs and hashtags. These new

Male Breast Cancer @MBCC_MHBT · 22 Apr 2017
Men carry #BRCA **mutations too.** @hessebiber @BRCAStudyBC **doing great work.** #MBCCFest17 #malebreastcancer #bcsm

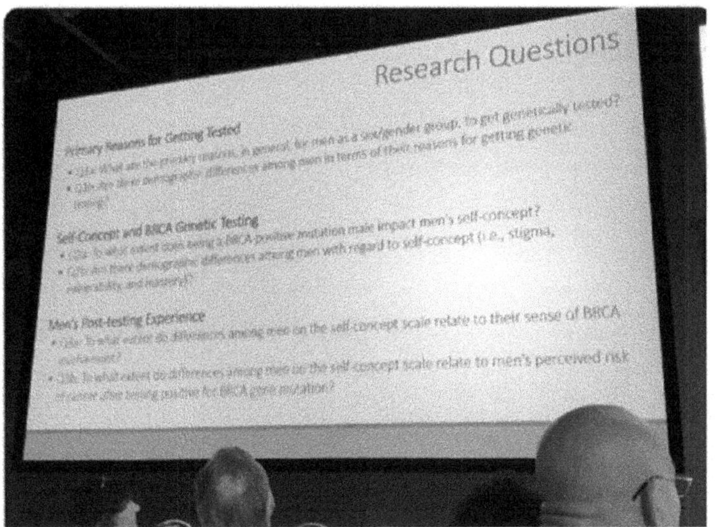

Figure 6.7 Non-storytelling tweet (1).

Prediction of #BreastCancer & #ProstateCancer Risks in Male #BRCA Carriers Using Polygenic Risk Scores #Genetics ncbi.nlm.nih.gov/m/pubmed/28448 ...

6:33 AM · 28 Apr 2017

Figure 6.8 Non-storytelling tweet (2).

Source: (URL to Lecarpentier et al., 2017).

markers, however, are more likely to prioritize content visibility and outreach over source visibility and author's stance. Shortened URLs, for instance, make space for more substantial tweet content while using multiple hashtags makes tweets retrievable by different "discourse communities" on the platform (Zappavigna, 2011).

Where authors engaged more explicitly with the external content they shared (i.e., in original tweets), interpretive dynamics surfaced more clearly (Figure 6.10). User 6, for instance, commented on the piece of news reported at the

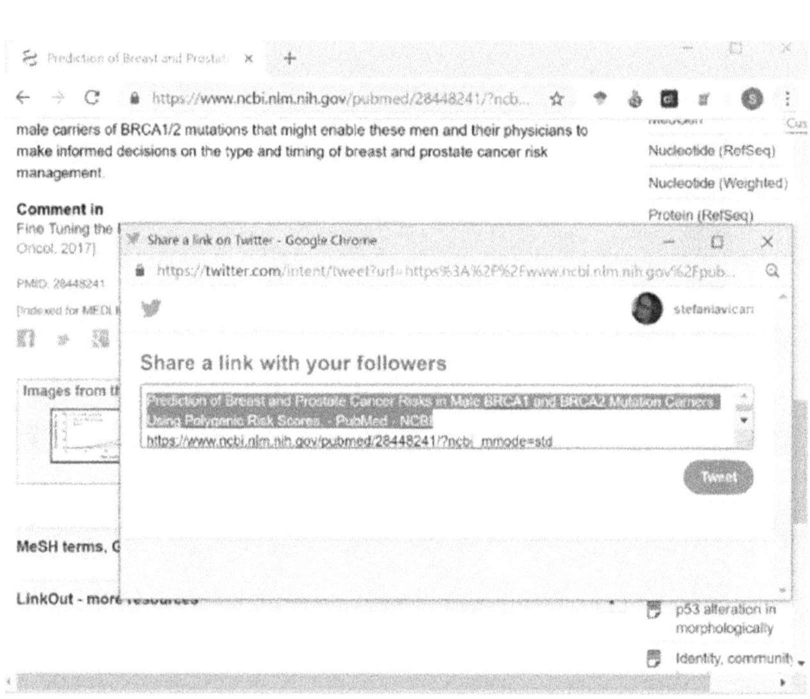

Figure 6.9 Button sharing generating the pre-modified version of the tweet of Figure 6.8.

#ICYMI: And surely companies will not use this piece of information to discriminate against people working for them ... 😔😔😔 #hcsm #bcsm #BRCA

mashable.com/2017/03/11/rep ...

Figure 6.10 Non-storytelling tweet (3) (anonymised and paraphrased).

Source: (URL to Begley, 2017).

tweeted URL, namely, a proposed bill that would allow companies in the US to collect genetic information from their employees.

The author used sarcasm to express their opinion about the bill by using the hashtag #ICYMI (i.e., "in case you missed it") and the repeated "pensive face" emoji. In this case, platform norms added to the effect of traditional markers of emotion (i.e., the ellipsis mark), providing additional and accentuating devices to express affect and attitudes.

In sum, my exploration of a month of BRCA content posted on Twitter in 2017 showed that both stories and non-stories are used by the BRCA public on the platform, with the former actually playing less of the central role described in previous digital and social media research. Both the topics and the sources of the stories and non-stories discussed in this section can give us a sense of the type of information, knowledge and expertise Twitter users draw upon to talk and learn about the BRCA mutations. Ultimately, this can also provide insight into the epistemic dynamics potentially emerging within the BRCA Twitter public, namely, into how Twitter users make sense of "BRCA". By bringing together the notions of social media issue publics, communities of practice and epistemic communities discussed in Chapters 2 and 4, the next section explores epistemic dynamics by focusing exactly on the content and the sources of information used by the BRCA Twitter public between 30 March and 29 April 2017.

Epistemics

Interest in epistemic dynamics has clearly emerged in research focused on "digital health platforms" (Lupton, 2014) or "experience exchange platforms" (Van Dijck et al., 2018) (see Chapter 7). As discussed earlier, investigations of mainstream platforms (e.g., Facebook, Twitter) seem instead to be primarily focusing on storytelling dynamics. Even in social media research, applying a Community of Practice (CoP) focus (see Chapter 4), the actual fabric of health-focused streams, that is, the potential combination of different types of knowledge within them, remains underexplored.

As we discussed in Chapter 2, with digital platforms becoming ubiquitous in everyday life, the concept of issue public has turned central to investigate the discursive work developed by social media users. The attention has been almost exclusively drawn to Twitter conversations about major events and breaking news, mostly overlooking mundane engagements with issues that are specifically central to the everyday of those involved. In other words, existing research tends to skim over the discursive work produced daily, in the absence of major events, by citizens engaging in discussions that directly resonate with their values, personal interests, and social groups (Krosnick, 1990).

The evolution of the BRCA public between 2013 and 2015 discussed in the earlier sections of this chapter shows, however, that Twitter is also populated by "resilient issue publics", that is, publics emerging and developing over time on the basis of their members' personal experience of the issue at stake, in conditions unrelated to emerging issues and acute events. The idea of "resilient issue public" is particularly relevant to health-centred social media threads because 1) health conditions are usually perceived as personal issues (Gonzalez-Polledo & Tarr, 2016), 2), health content is among the top searches on social media platforms (Pew Research Center, 2019) and 3) as discussed earlier, people use social media to connect with others in "illness subcultures" (Conrad et al., 2016).

Resilient and ad-hoc publics may temporarily intersect (see Figure 6.11), for instance, when a sudden event sheds light on an issue that is usually non-newsworthy (e.g., when a celebrity discloses information about a personal health condition), generating a peak of participation in the public debate about that specific issue. In other words, acute events throw ad-hoc publics into resilient ones. However, by investigating mundane and resilient (i.e., long-lived) rather than ad-hoc (i.e., heightened) conversations, we might be better placed to explore if and how contemporary social media platforms host epistemic dynamics comparable to those described in more traditional and enclosed online settings like dedicated forums, blogs or mailing lists (Akrich, 2010; Bellander & Landqvist, 2020) (see Chapter 3).

As shown in Figure 6.11, within resilient issue publics, CoPs might emerge, namely, "colocated or distributed" groups (Wenger et al., 2002, p. 25) might form, with their participants sharing personal understandings of shared issues (Lave & Wenger, 1991, p. 98). Some of these CoPs will focus almost

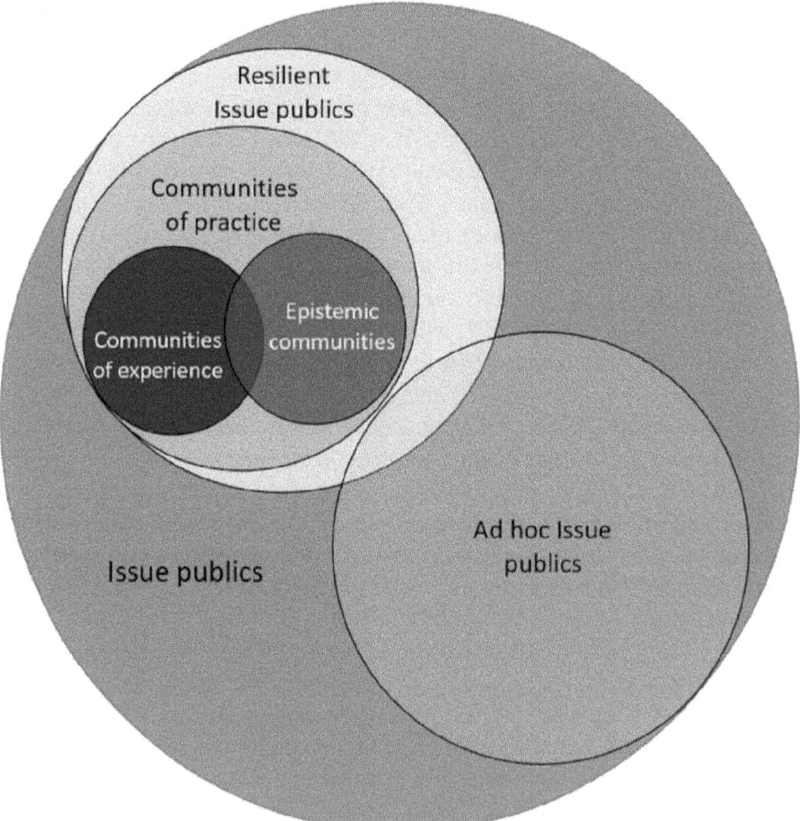

Figure 6.11 Issue publics, communities of practice and epistemic communities on social media.

exclusively on shared experience, primarily drawing upon experiential knowledge (see Akrich, 2010). Others will combine experiential and expert knowledge and evolve in "epistemic communities", that is, communities sharing argumentative resources combining lay (i.e., experiential) and scientific (i.e., credentialed) expertise and most likely to influence health policing (also see Haas, 1992, p. 3).

Sources of Information

The topics covered in the BRCA tweets discussed in the previous section focused on a range of themes, with strategies for risk assessment being the most frequent one, and genetic testing by far the most discussed strategy. As mentioned above, what often gets blurred in a microblogging environment like Twitter, and in its dynamics of intertextuality, is where the information being shared on the platform originates from. Figure 6.12 maps the sources of information explicitly referenced (e.g. via hyperlinks to external websites) in the

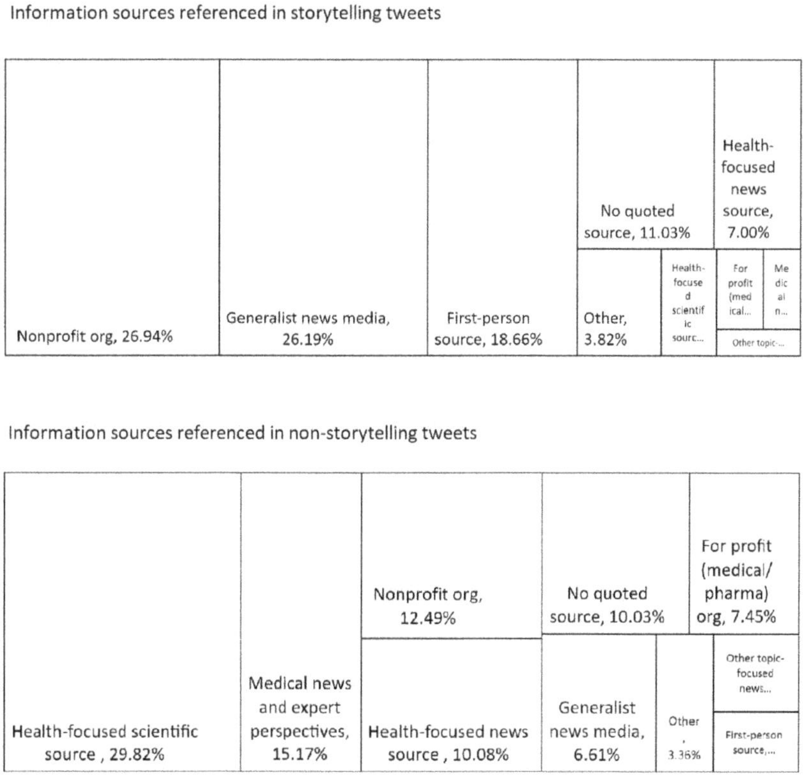

Figure 6.12 Sources of information in storytelling and non-storytelling tweets.

storytelling and non-storytelling tweets discussed in the previous section (for further information about the coding used in this phase of the research, please see Vicari, 2020).

Sources of Information in Storytelling Tweets

More than one fourth (i.e., 27%) of the storytelling tweets referenced non-profit organisation websites, with generalist news media being almost equally relevant (i.e., 26%). Among the top ten tweeters most often referencing these sources, five were advocacy organisations themselves (i.e., Facing Our Risk of Cancer Empowered, Male Breast Cancer Coalition, Men Have Breasts Too, National Hereditary Breast Cancer Helpline and Breast Advocate), with the rest being individual users. Again, this points to the centrality of "crowd-sourced storytelling" in contemporary advocacy action, as recently stressed by Trevisan: "Advocacy and activist groups . . . develop new techniques to influence public debate and policy decisions, using the Internet to crowd-source, organize, and disseminate their constituents' personal stories" (2017, p. 192).

Overall, in storytelling units referencing external sources, the voice of the individuals whose story was being told—that is, that of the initiators of these stories themselves—navigated different layers of mediation before reaching Twitter. In fact, it might not be surprising that Lesley Murphy's preventative mastectomy entered the Twittersphere via her blog (Figure 6.5), her Instagram account (Figure 6.2) and a number of generalist news media (e.g., *People*; see Stone, 2017). As a matter of fact, as a media celebrity, Murphy engages in daily self-branding tactics that require a certain level of personal disclosure and "context collapse" of social media activity (Khamis et al., 2017, p. 195). In my analysis, however, I soon realised that this ecological dimension also characterised the narration of ordinary citizens with extraordinary stories of health and illness. Louise Mallendar's story gives us a glimpse of this.

On 28 March 2017, Snow Elk Productions published a video on their YouTube channel for National Hereditary Breast Cancer Helpline (NHBCH) where Louise Mallendar recounts her story as a 36-year-old terminal cancer patient with BRCA 1 mutation (Snow Elk Productions, 2017).[4] In the video, Louise walks her audience through the different phases of her condition, describing both its impact on her family and her relationship with the medical information and the physicians involved in her diagnosis and treatment. The video first appeared in the dataset on 30 March in a retweet by an ordinary Twitter user and reappeared on 5, 6, 7, 8, 9 and 11 April, when it also got incorporated and commented on in an ITV news webpage (ITV News, 2017), quoted in a NHBCH tweet. The video reappeared on 12 and 13 April. On 15 April, NHBCH tweeted its own Facebook post announcing Louise's passing (Figure 6.13), being then retweeted by several BRCA patient advocates.

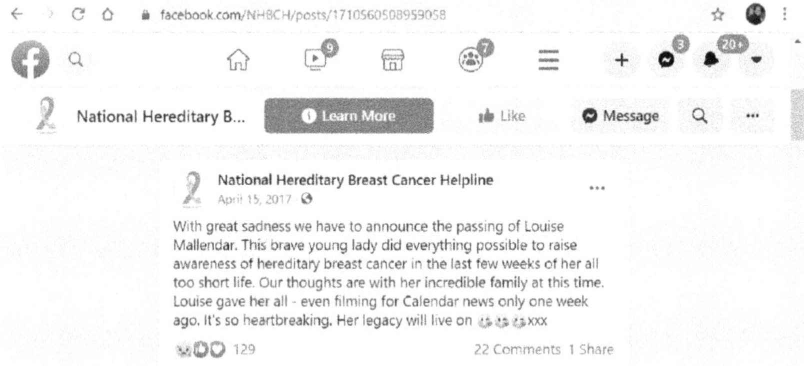

Figure 6.13 National Hereditary Breast Cancer Helpline announcing the passing of Louise Mallendar on Facebook.

Differently to Murphy's case, each digital artefact bringing Louise's story onto Twitter (i.e., video on Snow Elk Productions YouTube channel, piece on ITV news webpage, post on NHBCH Facebook page) played a different role in building BRCA awareness (and knowledge): Snow Elk Production's YouTube video—and its virality—made BRCA newsworthy, the piece on the ITV webpage widened BRCA visibility and the NHBCH Facebook post strengthened ties among BRCA advocates.

Sources of Information in Non-Storytelling Tweets

As shown in Figure 6.12, 45% of the tweets delivering non-storytelling content drew upon either traditional scientific sources or pieces reporting medical news and expert perspectives. This means that between 30 March 2017 and 29 April 2017, one third of the tweets reporting information relevant to the BRCA gene mutation as a health condition directly referenced traditional sources of medical expertise. The top four—and, overall, six out of the top ten—users most often referencing scientific sources, medical news or expert perspectives in their tweets were patient advocates with a substantial follower base and who "self-tagged" with a series of cancer and hereditary cancer hashtags (i.e., #bcsm, #BRCA, #breastcancer, #GenCSM, #genetictesting, #gyncsm, #hereditarycancer, #Lynchsyndrome, #NSGCgenepool and #PancChat) (Table 6.8). In fact, among the top ten, only one identified themselves as a medical doctor.

This clearly indicates that a number of individuals who would be traditionally identified as *lay* actors acted as key providers of scientific information within the BRCA resilient public on Twitter. In other words, their engagement with both the public and the platform translated into foregrounding their experiential knowledge but also acting as gatekeepers of traditional expert information.

Table 6.8 Top 4 users quoting scientific sources or medical news in the 2017 sample period.

Rank	*Author*	*Followers (04/2017)*	*Twitter bio (06/2019)*	*Evidence of patient advocacy*
1	Lisa M Guzzardi, RN	4,857	#PatientAdvocate providing up to date research for 3K+ consumers @ risk & clinicians #JournalClub #bcsm #gyncsm #PancChat #BRCA #hereditarycancer #NSGCgenepool	(Nawrat, 2019)
2	Amy Byer Shainman	4,909	Education—Advocacy—Support #BRCA #hereditarycancer—BRCA memoir now available—Speaker—Author—Producer @pinkandbluedoc @GenC_SM	(Byer Shainman, 2019)
3	Karen Lazarovitz	4,011	Creator #BRCA Sisterhood & Supportgroup #Montreal #breastcancer #hereditarycancer#genetictesting #publicspeaker my story #mastectomy #tattoos link below	(Kalinowicz, 2019)
4	Georgia Hurst	6,452	Mushrooms, microbes, and octopodes fascinate me. There's enough misery in the world, don't contribute to it. I miss Obama. #AmWriting #Lynchsyndrome#GenCSM.	(Hurst, 2019)

Conclusion: Six Propositions on Mainstream Social Media and Participatory Cultures of Health and Illness

Empirical work interested in the impact of social media usage on discursive practices in general, and participatory dynamics in particular, has drawn attention to the way social media sociotechnical infrastructures tend to destabilise traditional power roles in the construction of meaning around issues of public interest. This chapter has addressed these issues in relation to participatory dynamics focused on health and illness, specifically exploring curation, framing, storytelling, and epistemic practices.

The first part of the chapter focused on curation dynamics at two similar but temporarily distant time points in the life story of the BRCA Twitter public to unveil changes in platform functionality, that is, changes in the way Twitter use allowed or supported the coming to prominence of non-elite figures described in previous research (Bastos et al., 2012; Hermida, 2015; Jackson & Foucault Welles, 2015, 2016; Meraz & Papacharissi, 2013). We saw that between 2013 and 2015 in the BRCA Twitter public individual patient advocates supplanted advocacy organisations in top broadcasting and gatekeeping roles, with crowd-enabled replacing organisationally-enabled connective action (Bennett & Segerberg, 2013). In other words, not only did Twitter usage enhance the emergence of non-elite actors (Jackson & Foucault Welles, 2015, 2016; Meraz & Papacharissi, 2013) in the curation of BRCA topics, it also allowed the transfer of power roles from non-elite *collective* actors (i.e., advocacy organisations) to non-elite *individual* actors (i.e., patient advocates), that is, to minorities within minorities.

Shifts also occurred in the way in which the BRCA mutations were progressively framed as a health condition. In 2013, the BRCA Twitter public primarily relied upon content-based frames relevant to the Myriad Genetics' gene patents controversy. By February 2015, frames incorporated a range of specialist narratives: not only did they foreground breast cancer themes hardly present in mainstream representations of breast cancer (e.g., metastatic cancer); they drew links with similar but far less known hereditary cancer conditions (i.e., Lynch Syndrome). What remained unvaried in the BRCA stream between 2013 and 2015 was the temporary effect of heightened mainstream media exposure linked to Angelina Jolie's New York Times opinion pieces. In both occasions, the "Angelina effect" added a "hybrid" (Chadwick, 2013) dimension to the BRCA Twitter stream—a dimension where mainstream media shared gatekeeping prominence with non-elite actors. It probably also contributed to the emergence of BRCA-themed Twitter chats and, finally, foregrounded BRCA-related topics directly linked to the actress' experience of the BRCA condition. The hybrid dimension caused by the Angelina effect was, however, short-lived, with curation and framing dynamics occurring prior to Jolie's pieces resuming a few days after their publication.

The BRCA Twitter public also provides evidence that stories do matter, but they are not all that matters in social media health issue publics fed by and feeding into illness subcultures. The extensive informational practices analysed in this chapter were actually more likely to rely on non-storytelling information than on personal narratives and were highly shaped by and adapted to platform norms. Furthermore, when storytelling did appear, it was more often based on third-person narratives than on "self-stories" (Orgad, 2005).

The sources of information underlying storytelling and non-storytelling content shared within health issue publics on social media can give us a sense of the epistemic work developing within these publics. The "stories of others" discussed in this chapter were mainly borrowed from non-profit organisation websites and generalist news media for advocacy purposes (Trevisan, 2017). In other words, the voices of those living and initiating these stories—lay individuals with a BRCA story (Hardey, 2002)—travelled through different layers of mediation and became exemplar within the BRCA subculture. A large portion of non-narrative content directly referenced traditional scientific sources, with patient advocates acting as key providers of this content. While sharing features (e.g. their digital labour) with the health influencers described in previous research (McCosker, 2018), these individuals acted more as gatekeepers of scientific information than as social media "microcelebrities" (Abidin, 2016). They developed influence by regularly foregrounding selected sources of information rather than building a 360-degree persona "through empathy practices that sustain impactful connections" (McCosker, 2018, p. 4761).

Ultimately, the dynamics discussed in this chapter suggest a series of considerations about the relationship between mainstream social media and contemporary cultures of health and illness that I summarise as follows:

1. **The networked sociotechnical infrastructures provided by mainstream social media platforms certainly have an impact on the coming to prominence of citizens over traditional elite individuals (e.g., health professionals or policymakers), media (e.g., mainstream news outlets) and organisations (e.g., institutional health systems). This impact, however, intertwines with that of wider sociocultural dynamics**. The 1990s' progressive shift in the understanding of patienthood as an active form of engagement with health conditions—and the consequent emergence of the "active patients" described in Chapter 3—has certainly provided a fertile background for the development of personalised forms of engagement with topics related to health and illness. In the case of the BRCA mutations, rising public awareness around BRCA-related topics, also linked to the "Angelina effect", most likely also added to the development of personalised forms of engagement with these topics. Twitter's sociotechnical infrastructure, in particular its hosting specific networked curation and framing processes regulated by conversational and tagging markers, simply enhanced the *public* manifestation, and visibility, of these pre-existing or emerging personalised forms of engagement. It is then probably due to this combination of non-platform bound sociocultural dynamics and platform-specific sociotechnical infrastructures that,

in a two-year span, the public voice of individual patient advocates in the BRCA Twitter stream overcame that of traditional collective advocacy actors.

2. **The norms and conventions of social media platforms shape how information is shared and what becomes more visible in these sharing practices.** Twitter, for instance, is specifically designed in a way to foreground the visibility of tweeters and content, with less priority being given to the visibility of the sources of the information being shared in a tweet. For example, emojis add to traditional markers of expression (e.g. question marks) while hashtags enhance outreach, that is, they make it possible for content to be easily reached by users interested in specific topics. The platform's markers of reference (e.g. shortened URLs as opposed to traditional citations), however, while constantly evolving (e.g., from "via" used in the past to new referencing systems) do not necessarily make it easy to assess the quality of the information source from which the content being shared comes from.
3. **Social media's functionalities for resilient (i.e., long-lasting) health issue publics, and the illness subcultures they may represent, can vary highly over time.** For the BRCA public, for instance, in April-June 2013 the platform worked primarily as an organisation-centred "news reporting mechanism" (Papacharissi, 2012), focusing on events happening on the ground. In February-April 2015, these dynamics had been overturned by the emergence of BRCA-related content characterised by specialist topical dimensions. In this second scenario, Twitter worked then more as a crowdsourced specialist "awareness system" (Hermida, 2010, p. 298) that helped those involved in the BRCA Twitter public make sense of a range of dimensions characterising the experience of living with a BRCA mutation.
4. **Contrary to what happens in more dedicated and often contained digital spaces (e.g. user lists, patient or carer blogs or forums), most mainstream social media also allow users to participate in health issue publics without having to disclose their "personal commitment" (Akrich, 2010) to the issue at stake or their self-story related to it.** This openness allows and legitimises loose forms of participation in health issue publics and illness subcultures, offering means of engagement for those unwilling to share personal narratives or strongly and/or publicly commit to advocacy or activist action.
5. **Mainstream social media platforms allow for "experiential" and "expert" knowledge to easily intersect in health issue publics, often enhancing extensive epistemic work.** This happens in varied forms of mediated and unmediated discourse practices that incorporate both storytelling and non-storytelling content, with traditional scientific information becoming an important element of the latter.
6. **At the heart of the intersection of experiential and expert knowledge are often "lay experts", namely, individuals experiencing the condition**

discussed within the issue public, without necessarily having professional scientific training. These lay experts can become exemplars and/or act as gatekeepers of scientific information within the health issue public and the wider illness subculture. For instance, in this chapter we saw that in 2017, Louise Mallendar became an exemplar while Lisa Guizzardi acted as a gatekeeper for the BRCA Twitter public and the wider BRCA illness subculture.

Notes

1. I only refer to original Twitter handles of, and content posted by, organisations, public figures, journalists, news editors, or individuals who have publicly spoken of their engagement with BRCA advocacy outside Twitter or given me their consent to disclose their Twitter handle as part of the study. Where none of the abovementioned conditions were met, handles are replaced with pseudonyms (e.g. Individual x) and tweets paraphrased.
2. Lynch Syndrome is an inherited cancer syndrome derived from a genetic mutation that, like BRCA1 and BRCA2, increases the risk of different types of cancer at a young age (Genetic and Rare Disease Information Center, 2021).
3. To reproduce the original vernacular of anonymised tweets, I created a fictional Twitter account with handle 'User x' and posted the paraphrased tweets on the platform, setting this content as not publicly available. This chapter presents screengrabs of these tweets.
4. The video is available at: www.youtube.com/watch?v=hEU8IzGUmv4.

Reference List

Abidin, C. (2016). "Aren't these just young, rich women doing vain things online?": Influencer selfies as subversive frivolity. *Social Media + Society*, *2*(2), 2056305116641342.

Akrich, M. (2010). From communities of practice to epistemic communities: Health mobilizations on the internet. *Sociological Research Online*, *15*(2), 1–17.

Barton, A. (2013, October 3). Canada's hereditary-cancer clinics feel the Angelina effect. *The Globe and Mail*. www.theglobeandmail.com

Bastos, M., Galdini Raimundo, R. L., & Travitzki, R. (2012). Gatekeeping Twitter: Message diffusion in political hashtags. *Media, Culture & Society*, *35*(2), 260–270.

Begley, S. (2017, March 11). Republican bill would let employers demand workers' get genetic testing. *Mashable*. https://mashable.com/2017/03/11/republicans-genetic-tests-employers/?europe=true

Bellander, T., & Landqvist, M. (2020). Becoming the expert constructing health knowledge in epistemic communities online. *Information, Communication & Society*, *23*(4), 507–522.

Benkler, Y. (2006). *The wealth of networks: How social production transforms markets and freedom*. Yale University Press.

Bennett, W. L., & Segerberg, A. (2013). *The logic of connective action: Digital media and the personalization of contentious politics*. Cambridge University Press.

Bennett, W. L., Segerberg, A., & Walker, S. (2014). Organization in the crowd: Peer production in large-scale networked protests. *Information, Communication & Society*, *17*(2), 232–260.

Bers, M. U. (2009). New media for new organs: A virtual community for paediatric post: Transplant patients. *Convergence*, *15*(4), 462–469.

Borzekowski, D. L. G., Guan, Y. G., Smith, K. C., Erby, L. H., & Roter, D. L. (2014). The Angelina effect: Immediate reach, grasp, and impact of going public. *Genetics in Medicine*, *16*, 516–521.

Bruns, A., & Burgess, J. E. (2011). The use of Twitter hashtags in the formation of ad hoc publics. In *Proceedings of the 6th European Consortium for Political Research (ECPR) General Conference*, Reykjavik, Iceland.

Bruns, A., & Burgess, J. E. (2012). Researching news discussion on Twitter: New methodologies. *Journalism Studies*, *13*, 801–814.

Bury, M. (1982). Chronic illness as biographical disruption. *Sociology of Health & Illness*, *4*(2), 167–182.

Bury, M. (2001). Illness narratives: Fact or fiction? *Sociology of Health & Illness*, *23*(3), 263–285.

Byer Shainman, A. (2019). Amy Byer Shainman. *FORCE*. www.facingourrisk.org/get-involved/how-to-help/volunteer-fundraise/volunteer-spotlight/amy-byer-shainman.php

Carmody, C., & Sartor, A. (2013, April 15). Human gene patents are wrong: That's all there is to it! *Breast Cancer Action*. https://bcaction.org/2013/04/15/human-gene-patents-are-wrong-thats-all-there-is-to-it/

Chadwick, A. (2013). *The hybrid media system: Politics and power*. Oxford University Press.

Cohen, J. H., & Raymond, J. M. (2011). How the internet is giving birth (to) a new social order. *Information, Communication & Society*, *14*(6), 937–957.

Conrad, P., Bandini, J., & Vasquez, A. (2016). Illness and the Internet: From private to public experience. *Health*, *20*(1), 22–32.

Dean, M. (2016). Celebrity health announcements and online health information seeking: An analysis of Angelina Jolie's preventative health decision. *Health Communication*, *31*(6), 752–761.

Dunlop, K., Kirk, J., & Tucker, K. (2014). In the wake of Angelina: Managing a family history of breast cancer. *Australian Family Physician*, *43*, 76–78.

Evans, D., Barwell, J., Eccles, D. M., Collins, A., Izatt, L., Jacobs, C., . . . Murray, A. (2014). The Angelina Jolie effect: How high celebrity profile can have a major impact on provision of cancer related services. *Breast Cancer Research*, *16*, article 442.

Frohlich, D. O., & Zmyslinski-Seelig, A. N. (2016). How Uncover Ostomy challenges ostomy stigma, and encourages others to do the same. *New media & society*, *18*(2), 220–238.

Genetic and Rare Disease Information Center. (2021). *Lynch syndrome*. https://rarediseases.info.nih.gov/. Retrieved 18 June 2021.

Gonzalez-Polledo, E. (2016). Chronic media worlds: Social media and the problem of pain communication on Tumblr. *Social Media + Society*, *2*(1), 2056305116628887.

Gonzalez-Polledo, E., & Tarr, J. (2016). The thing about pain: The remaking of illness narratives in chronic pain expressions on social media. *New Media & Society*, *18*(8), 1455–1472.

Haas, P. M. (1992). Introduction: Epistemic communities and international policy coordination. *International Organization*, 1–35.

Hardey, M. (2002). "The story of my illness": Personal accounts of illness on the Internet. *Health*, *6*(1), 31–46.

Hermida, A. (2010). Twittering the news. *Journalism Practice*, *4*(3), 297–308.

Hermida, A. (2015). Power plays on social media. *Social Media + Society*, *1*(1), 2056305115580340.

Hurst, G. (2019, February 26). Living Scan to Scan with Lynch Syndrome. *Cure*. www.curetoday.com. Retrieved 18 June 2021.

Hydén, L. C. (1997). Illness and narrative. *Sociology of Health & Illness*, *19*(1), 48–69.

ITV News (2017, April 10). *Chesterfield mum, 36, with terminal breast cancer raises awareness of faulty gene*. www.ITV.com/news/calendar/2017-04-10/mother-36-with-terminal-breast-cancer-raises-awareness-of-faulty-gene/

Jackson, S., & Foucault Welles, B. (2015). Hijacking #myNYPD: Social media dissent and networked counterpublics. *Journal of Communication*, *65*, 932–952.

Jackson, S., & Foucault Welles, B. (2016). #Ferguson is everywhere: Initiators in emerging counterpublic networks. *Information, Communication & Society*, *19*(3), 397–418.

Jolie, A. (2013, May 4). My medical choice. *The New York Times*. www.nytimes.com

Jolie, A. (2015, March 24). Angelina Jolie pitt: Diary of a surgery. *The New York Times*. www.nytimes.com

Kalinowicz, M. (2019, January 8). Montrealer says breast implants banned in Europe still being used in Canada. *Global News*. https://globalnews.ca

Kamenova, K., Reshef, A., & Caulfield, T. (2014). Angelina Jolie's faulty gene: Newspaper coverage of a celebrity's preventive bilateral mastectomy in Canada, the United States, and the United Kingdom. *Genetics in Medicine*, *16*, 522–528.

Khamis, S., Ang, L., & Welling, R. (2017). Self-branding, "micro-celebrity" and the rise of social media influencers. *Celebrity Studies*, *8*(2), 191–208.

Klawiter, M. (1999). Racing for the cure, walking women, and toxic touring: Mapping cultures of action within the Bay Area terrain of breast cancer. *Social Problems*, *46*(1), 104–126.

Kluger, J., Park, A., Pickert, K., Schrobsdorff, S., Sifferlin, A., & Rothman, L. (2013, May 27). The Angelina effect. *Time*, *181*(20), 28–34.

Kosenko, K. A., Binder, A., & Hurley, R. (2016). Celebrity influence and identification: A test of the Angelina effect. *Journal of Health Communication*, *21*(3), 318–326.

Koster, S. (2017, April, 14). *Blessed to be BRCA aware. Hi my name is Sarah, I'm 31 and I'm BRCA 1. Medium*. https://medium.com/@sazkoster/blessed-to-be-brca-aware-269df2755bf3

Krosnick, J. A. (1990). Government policy and citizen passion: A study of issue publics in contemporary America. *Political Behavior*, *12*(I), 59–92.

Lave, J., & Wenger, E. (1991). *Situated learning: Legitimate peripheral participation*. Cambridge University Press.

Lecarpentier, J., Silvestri, V., Kuchenbaecker, K. B., Barrowdale, D., Dennis, J., McGuffog, L., . . . Tischkowitz, M. (2017). Prediction of breast and prostate cancer risks in male BRCA1 and BRCA2 mutation carriers using polygenic risk scores. *Journal of Clinical Oncology*, *35*(20), 2240.

Lupton, D. (2014). The commodification of patient opinion: The digital patient experience economy in the age of big data. *Sociology of Health & Illness*, *36*(6), 856–869.

Lupton, D. (2017). Introduction. In Lupton, D. (Ed.) *Digitised health, medicine and risk* (pp. 1–3). Routledge.

McCormick, S., Brown, P., & Zavestoski, S. (2003). The personal is scientific, the scientific is political: The public paradigm of the environmental breast cancer movement. *Sociological Forum*, *18*(4), 545–576.

McCosker, A. (2018). Engaging mental health online: Insights from beyondblue's forum influencers. *New Media & Society*, *20*(12), 4748–4764.

Mehta, S. (2013, November 17). Oncologists warn of Angelina Jolie effect. *Times of India*. http://timesofindia.indiatimes.com

Meraz, S., & Papacharissi, Z. (2013). Networked gatekeeping and networked framing on #Egypt. *The International Journal of Press/Politics*, *18*(2), 138–166.

Murphy, L. (2017). Breaking up with my breasties: The naked truth. In *The road les traveled*. https://theroadlestraveled.com

Myrick, J. G., Holton, A. E., Himelboim, I., & Love, B. (2016). # Stupidcancer: Exploring a typology of social support and the role of emotional expression in a social media community. *Health communication*, *31*(5), 596–605.

National Cancer Institute at the National Institutes of Health (NCI) (2021). *BRCA1 and BRCA2: Cancer risk and genetic testing*. www.cancer.gov. Retrieved 18 June 2021.

Nawrat, A. (2019, July 2). Oncology: Ten of the leading influencers in the field. *Pharmaceutical Technology*. www.pharmaceutical-technology.com

Neporent, L. (2013, October 15). Jolie's doctor says her story raises awareness, saves lives. *ABC News*. http://abcnews.go.com

Noar, S. M., Althouse, B. M., Ayers, J. W., Francis, D. B., & Ribisi, K. M. (2015). Cancer information seeking in the digital age: Effects of Angelina Jolie's prophylactic mastectomy announcement. *Medical Decision Making*, *35*, 16–21.

Orgad, S. (2005). *Storytelling online: Talking breast cancer on the Internet*. Peter Lang.

Papacharissi, Z. (2016). Affective publics and structures of storytelling: Sentiment, events and mediality. *Information, Communication & Society*, *19*(3), 307–324.

Papacharissi, Z., & de Fatima Oliveira, M. (2012). Affective news and networked publics: The rhythms of news storytelling on #Egypt. *Journal of Communication*, *62*, 266–282.

Pew Research Center. (2019). *In emerging economies, smartphone and social media users have broader social networks*. https://www.pewresearch.org/internet/2019/08/22/social-activities-information-seeking-on-subjects-like-health-and-education-top-the-list-of-mobile-activities/

Rogers, R. (2019). *Doing digital methods*. Sage.

Snow Elk Production (2017). *NHBCH: Louise's legacy: "Make one person aware"*. www.youtube.com/watch?v=hEU8IzGUmv4

Song, S., Zhao, Y. C., Yao, X., Ba, Z., & Zhu, Q. (2021, June, 24). Short video apps as a health information source: An investigation of affordances, user experience and users' intention to continue the use of TikTok. *Internet Research*. https://www.emerald.com/insight/content/doi/10.1108/INTR-10-2020-0593/full/html

Stone, N. (2017, April 14). *Bachelor* alum lesley murphy undergoes preventative double mastectomy nearly 3 years following her mother's breast cancer diagnosis. *People*. https://people.com/tv/bachelor-alum-lesley-murphy-undergoes-preventative-double-mastectomy-breast-cancer/

Tanis, M. (2008). Health-related online forums: What's the big attraction? *Journal of Health Communication*, *13*(7), 698–714.

Trevisan, F. (2016). *Disability rights advocacy online: Voice, empowerment and global connectivity*. Routledge.

Trevisan, F. (2017). Crowd: Sourced advocacy: Promoting disability rights through online storytelling. *Public Relations Inquiry*, *6*(2), 191–208.

Tucker, K. I. (2016). Watch out men, breast cancer gene can get you too. *Forward*. https://forward.com/culture/347346/watch-out-men-breast-cancer-gene-can-get-you-too/

Van Dijck, J., Poell, T., & de Waal, M. (2018). *The platform society: Public values in a connective world*. Oxford University Press.

Vicari, S. (2017). Twitter and non-elites: Interpreting power dynamics in the life story of the (#) BRCA Twitter stream. *Social Media + Society*, *3*(3), 2056305117733224.

Vicari, S. (2020). Is it all about storytelling? Living and learning hereditary cancer on Twitter. *New Media and Society*, 1461444820926632.

Wenger, E., McDermott, R. A., & Snyder, W. (2002). *Cultivating communities of practice: A guide to managing knowledge*. Harvard business press.

Zappavigna, M. (2011). Ambient affiliation: A linguistic perspective on Twitter. *New Media & Society*, *13*(5), 788–806.

7 Participatory Cultures of Health and Illness on Digital Health Platforms

Introduction

In 2020, the International Telecommunication Union (ITU) and World Health Organization (WHO) published the "Digital Health Platform" handbook. The manuscript was developed in the context of the "Be Healthy, Be Mobile" digital health initiative, with the aim of proving a toolkit "to help countries create a digital health platform (DHP) to serve as the underlying infrastructure for an interoperable and integrated national digital health system" (ITU & WTO, p. v). Perfectly embracing a vision of Information and Communication Technologies (ICTs) as empowering agents (see Chapter 4), this publication is indicative of the current global push towards integrating digital health initiatives into national public health and care services. The handbook itself frames these initiatives as necessarily shaped by a "platform concept design approach", namely, "linking together disparate and unconnected systems and applications", "thinking holistically and flexibly", using "seamless interoperability" and increasingly working as "underlying infrastructure[s]" (ITU & WTO, p. v).

As a matter of fact, the WTO and ITU's Digital Health Platform handbook defines digital health platforms in institutionalised, infrastructural and holistic terms as regional-level, centralised health information infrastructures to which external applications, ranging from software programs, digital tools and patient-engagement apps, link to support healthcare delivery (ITU & WTO, p. v). The "platform concept" these institutionalised and infrastructural super platforms are said to exploit is then predominantly focused on technical affordances and on their potential for public health and care services.

While the Digital Health Platform handbook provides an extremely topical picture of the role and potential impact increasingly ascribed to digital health platforms, it falls short in giving a sense of the current constellation of digital health platforms employed across contexts, markets, communities and use purposes. Perhaps most importantly, it also fails to acknowledge the existence of a "politics of platforms" (Gillespie, 2010; Hands, 2013), namely of a wide set of implications characterising the mainstreaming of digital platforms in everyday lives. As discussed in Chapter 2, the "platform concept" developed within the field of platform studies situates computational or, more broadly,

DOI: 10.4324/9780429469145-10

technical affordances, within political, economic, and social systems, "where software processes, patterns of information circulation, communicative practices, social practices, and political contexts are articulated with and redefined by each other in complex ways" (Langlois et al., 2009, p. 416). Looked at from this perspective, digital health platforms work through a number of interlinking dimensions—computational, political, figurative and architectural—that challenge the "technical neutrality and progressive openness" (Gillespie, 2010, p. 360) rhetoric adopted to promote and shape initiatives like the Digital Health Platform handbook.

After introducing a tentative and fluid typology of digital health platforms, the chapter develops through two main parts. First, it presents a discussion of the political economy of digital health platforms, focusing on its implications for the emergence or hindering of participatory cultures of health and illness. Then, it shifts the focus to everyday experiences of digital health to investigate how and to what extent users "resist" structures and norms embedded in the very design and rationale of most contemporary digital health platforms.

Digital Health Platforms

The term "digital health platform" has come to indicate a varied range of websites, digital applications and devices used within practices related to health and/or illness. We might attempt to build a typology of platforms based on the primary purpose ascribed to them by their providers. A first category is that of *tracking platforms*, which are primarily used to track and monitor a person's physical performance (e.g., Fitbit, Map my run and 30 Days fitness at home), lifestyle (e.g., ShopWell: Better Food Choices, Health and Nutrition Guide & Fitness Calculators) or health condition (e.g., Flaredown, MyIBDcare) (Jewell, 2020a, 2020b; Weinberg, 2020). Overlapping with tracking platforms are *self-diagnosis platforms*—specifically meant to help users self-diagnose symptoms or conditions (e.g., Sintomate, WebMD, 23andme) (The Medical Futurist, 2019). *Patient experience exchange platforms* used to be a separate category of platforms exclusively meant to build patients' social networks and data exchanges (e.g., PLM) (Wicks et al., 2010)—services that, however, are now offered by most digital health platforms. Finally, a less investigated and yet extremely interesting category is that of *feedback platforms*, which offer services dedicated to providing feedback about patients' experiences of health and social care services (e.g. Care Opinion) (Petrakaki, 2021). This brief typology, while certainly not exhaustive, gives a sense of the proliferation of opportunities brought by digital health platforms for people to seek and share health information with lay users or health professionals, but also to store and diarise their own biometric data.

A growing body of work developing at the intersection of science and technology studies, political economy, and the sociology of health and illness is increasingly investigating digital health platforms beyond their technical dimension and affordances. On the one hand, studies are focusing on their political economy and its impact on users, values, and public health systems (e.g., Van Dijck & Poell, 2016). On the other, work is exploring these platforms as sociocultural artefacts experienced and shaped by users in and across contexts (e.g., Lupton, 2014a, 2017a). The remainder of the chapter will draw upon work from each of these research strands to further explore how digital health platforms relate to contemporary cultures of health and illness.

The Political Economy of Digital Health Platforms

In many ways, and through different business solutions, digital health platforms capitalise on the digital and health participatory drives that we historicised in Chapters 2 and 3. Common promotional rhetoric thrives on the promise to offer personalised answers to health questions while simultaneously helping the public good via "participatory practices", "patient engagement" and "data openness" (Van Dijck & Poell, 2016). Underlying these and similar claims is the idea that digital health platforms, while embracing the contemporary push towards personalised medicine (see Chapter 4), have a positive societal impact. Platforms are often promoted as means to build new ways to connect with others and develop via data sharing practices. These practices are themselves framed as altruistic, oriented to the public good, and part of a new "moral economy" (Fotopoulou, 2018). To explore and challenge these claims, the following five sections will each discuss one aspect characterising contemporary digital health platforms: the commodification of patients' data, the dataist turn in self-tracking and monitoring practices, the often-ephemeral openness of "open data" in proprietary systems, the infrastructural turn of giant tech companies and the emergence of transient forms of citizenship. While looking at them separately, we will highlight the intersections and recursive relationships between these aspects. Each section will focus on one aspect by zooming in on one specific digital health platform (i.e., 23andMe, Fitbit, PatientsLikeMe, ParkinsonMPower, and Care Opinion). Not only will this allow us to explore the heterogeneous politico-economic landscape of digital health platforms and its implications for the development of specific cultures of health and illness; it will also lay the grounds for the remainder of the chapter to focus on the different forms of "data labour" emerging on digital health platforms.

The Unbalanced "Gift Exchange" in the Commodification of Patient Data

23andme, arguably the largest commercial direct-to-consumer DNA testing service available on the market, provides a meaningful example of a typical promotional rhetoric adopted by digital health platforms. At the time of writing, 23andme's website uses its homepage to remind you that "DNA insights are an essential part of *your health picture*." This reminder sets the grounds to help you self-acknowledge that "You are already doing so much to track your health" and invite you to "Add *personalised DNA insights* for a more complete picture of your health". Scrolling down the page, you are then prompted to

> Know you're making a difference. When you opt in to participate in our research, you join forces with millions of other people contributing to science. Your *participation* could help lead to discoveries that may one day make an *impact* on your own health, the health of your family and ultimately, *people around the world.*
>
> (Look at you go.) (23andme, 2021, emphasis added)

Drawing upon Tutton's (2002) work on "gift relationships" in genetics research, Harris and colleagues (2013) discuss 23andme's model of company-consumer relationship as based on a "gift exchange" that blurs commercial transactions and financial beneficiaries by exploiting participatory narratives and digital playfulness. Let us see how this works in practice. 23andme consumers, when sending their saliva sample to the company, pay for the sample to be analysed and for a report to be sent back to them. With the purchase of this service they are however also invited to sign a consent form that allows the company to store the sample's genomic data and exercise proprietary claims on them, ultimately transferring the rights to any financial gain from future research to the company (Harris et al., 2013; Van Dijck & Poell, 2016).

In the process, consumers are then given the chance to "participate" in research and benefit the wider community. "Participation", however, here primarily means waiving personal data ownership. Not only do consumers "gift" their genomic information; they are also nudged to share additional personal information via fun surveys and interactive features (Saukko, 2018, p. 1318; Van Dijck & Poell, 2016, p. 3). Saukko describes this as "a flow-inducing experience of wandering along and getting lost in exploring different paths, companionship and conversations" (2018, p. 1318). In sum, this experience is designed in a way to engage and connect consumers in a prolonged and enjoyable immersion. Ultimately, for the consumer, the gift exchange enhanced in their starting a relationship with 23andme translates into "*intangible benefits* such as enhanced self-worth, enhanced reputation, a sense of public good, personal satisfaction and the prospect of reward or reciprocity" (Harris et al., 2013, p. 245 emphasis added). For the company, it results in the financial benefits deriving from the commodification of consumers' data, in what Lupton (2014b) defines as the "digital patient experience economy". In this economy, individuals' experiences of health and illness acquire a commercial value that directly benefits those hosting and aggregating data sharing practices, namely, digital health platform providers.

Self-, Social- and Panoptic Surveillance in Market Driven Dataist Systems

Part of Google LLC multinational corporation, Fitbit is an American consumer electronics and fitness company that offers a range of self-tracking wearable devices. During the third quarter of 2020, Fitbit ranked among the top five companies in the global wearable market, against a background marked by a general market surge due to the Covid-19 pandemic (IDC, 2020). Fitbit use involves wearing a device that monitors and records one or more activities (e.g., walking, burning calories, sleeping) and connecting to a personalised interface—through the Fitbit website or app—to upload the data recorded by the device to a cloud-based system. Users can access activity reports and track their data over time or compare them to those of other Fitbit users. They can also enter other personal information, for instance, about their food consumption or mood (see Fotopoulou & O'Riordan, 2017, pp. 55–56). In 2018, the company launched "Fitbit Care", a product combining self-tracking and monitoring services with a series of personalised digital interventions (e.g., groups, challenges, workouts) aimed at managing health issues (Charitsis, 2019).

Fitbit can be seen as perfectly integrated in the framework of the "quantified self" daily routine. Coined in 2007 by Wired journalists Gary Wolf and Kevin Kelly, the "quantified self" term has come to address the mundane work of self-trackers, namely individuals who engage with daily uses of digital technologies to monitor and measure themselves (Lupton, 2016). Members of the official "Quantified Self movement" organise and attend meet-ups and conferences, and populate online forums (Nafus & Sherman, 2014). The main activity here is that of discussing the value of self-tracking in everyday life, or of "self-knowledge through numbers", as the movement's original tagline went (Schüll, 2018, p. 27). The Quantified Self website provides extensive information on how to get involved in "an international community of users and makers of self-tracking tools" (Quantified Self, 2021). Since Wolf and Kelly's initiative, the Quantified Self idea has gained traction among a wide range of users differently engaged with self-tracking and self-monitoring practices, whether or not involved in the official Quantified Self movement. This drive has, of course, also attracted an increasing number of digital entrepreneurs, bolstering the development of self-tracking platforms. Fitbit can be seen as representative of these platforms.

The "Fitbit model" integrates "private self-tracking" with "communal self-tracking" (Lupton, 2016). In other words, Fitbit users use wearable devices to track their own personal data but they are also encouraged to share these data to pursue a sort of "community development". Lupton (2016) defines self-tracking activities like those happening via Fitbit as "dataveillance, or the watching of people using technologies that generate data", with this watching having a much broader and undefined reach than that typical of traditional surveillance systems (Van Dijck, 2014). Hence, data generated on and by self-tracking devices like Fitbit may have a longer life than that expected by wearable users (and original data owners): they can be repurposed in different contexts and/or be at the centre of financial transitions, as we discussed in the last section. While private self-tracking is an expression of self-surveillance, communal self-tracking can be seen as a form of social surveillance, namely, of watching others and being watched in panoptic dynamics (Marwick, 2012). Thus, in generating a continuous intertwining of dataveillance dynamics, Fitbit self-tracking affordances blur private and public, domestic and communal domains, with the acts of watching and being watched informing self-discipline and impression management. In monitoring themselves and each other, users formulate views of what is normal, or average in the community, "creating an internalized gaze that contextualizes appropriate behavior" (Marwick, 2012, p. 384).

In fact, while promoting cultures of dataveillance, Fitbit invites users to confront themselves with their own personal information and to engage with this information to improve their lives. Drawing upon Foucault's conceptualisation of "biopower" (2019), Fotopoulou and O'Riordan (2017) define Fitbit's self-tracking system as constructing a "biopedagogy", namely, as building a set of normative assumptions about how one should live, and about their responsibility with regards to their behaviour to maintain or achieve good health. As Esmonde and Jette put it: the "Idealized Fitbit subjects take walks or engage in other activities throughout the day to increase their step count, always reach (at least) 10,000 steps, and prioritize their health through an engagement with risk-minimizing behaviours" (2020, p. 301). On Fitbit, social surveillance evolves from Marwick's (2012) conceptualisations: not only do users monitor themselves and each other and assess what is normal and average in the community; they also measure their performance against a higher target formulated by Fitbit itself. As a matter of fact, in the context of Fitbit's biopedagogy, "self-responsible users" actually exert very limited individual agency outside the "acceptable modes of conduct [set by] a neoliberal health landscape" (Fotopoulou & O'Riordan, 2017, p. 65). This neoliberal landscape is firmly grounded in objective understandings of health and illness, constructed via the quantification of self through data and quantified methods, so-called "dataism" (van Dijck, 2014).

Yet, how does "dataism" talk to the dynamics of lay expertise and experiential knowledge that we discussed in previous chapters (see Chapters 3 and 6)? In their analysis of Fitbit use, Fotopoulou and O'Riordan (2017, p. 66) provide an extremely relevant consideration:

> We may consequently think of a diffraction of expertise: from platforms (that set the protocols of health), through to bodies (that generate data in compliance with these protocols), back through the platforms (that provide the interpretation of the data); a recursive loop that opens up more markets for devices that track data.

This "diffraction of expertise" is entirely designed, regulated and measured through platform-driven, and most often market-driven, dataist systems. As such, it seems to leave very little room for the experiential and embodied knowledge that we discussed earlier as potentially providing participatory and activist means of resistance for individuals and patients.

"Data Openness" in Proprietary Systems?

At the time of writing, PatientsLikeMe (PLM) is among the most studied Western digital health platforms, with a quick search on Google Scholar returning

7,880 academic articles mentioning it. PLM is a for-profit organisation founded in 2004 by Jamie and Ben Heywood, following their brother Stephen's diagnosis with Amyotrophic lateral sclerosis (ALS). According to PLM's website, the Heywood brothers ultimately realised that what they should be looking for in their efforts to help find a cure for ALS—or ways to improve life through it—was the "aggregated real-world experiences of others living with and fighting to survive ALS" (PLM, 2021). In fact, PLM is now a health information sharing website in use by individuals tracking and sharing everyday personal information (e.g., symptoms, medication, participation in clinical trials) about one or more among 2,800 health conditions.

PLM then presents itself as a platform enhancing the emergence of illness-based "patient communities" and ultimately mediating relationships between different health stakeholders, ranging from patients and their families, to health professionals, pharmaceutical companies, research bodies and nongovernmental organizations. What could probably be seen as the most revolutionary idea behind PLM as a digital health platform is the premise that unsupervised and self-reported experiences can become evidence for clinical research, along with traditional scientific and medical data (Kallinikos & Tempini, 2014). In 2010, for instance, the PLM ALS patient community started to self-track their use of lithium carbonate on the platform. This PLM-organised and patient self-administered trial was meant to test the hypothesis—advanced by a group of Italian scientists—that the drug slowed the progression of the disease. Preliminary results of the study were made available after nine months, refuting the hypothesis that lithium carbonate had any positive effects on ALS patients (Wicks et al., 2011). Conventional clinical trials later confirmed these results.

It is important to highlight that it is not uncommon for patients with rare or incurable diseases to experiment with drugs that have not yet received regulatory approval but have shown potential in preliminary research. What however was new in this case is that PLM provided a platform for patients to track and share data about their self-experimentation and for these data to be aggregated and analysed in an "observational environment" and using standardised scales. Former PLM Research and Development Director Paul Wicks and colleagues have countered accusations of a general lack of validity of trials outside traditional clinical protocols arguing that observational studies like that conducted by PLM with its ALS patient community should not be seen as apt to replace traditional clinical trials but might "be useful for accelerating clinical discovery and evaluating the effectiveness of drugs already in use" (Wicks et al., 2011, p. 411).

It is hard to deny that patients did play a central role in the ALS observational study just described. For those who took part in the study, "participation" meant deciding to try lithium carbonate and being willing to track, monitor and share information about their use of the drug and perceived effects of it in what Lupton (2016) would define as "self-tracking citizenship', namely a communal self-tracking experience. There is a strong sense of agency in this choice, one most likely based on lived experiences of the disease and of the time (Charmaz, 1991), or lack of it, to find treatments. This agency was certainly exerted to produce change that may benefit the individual engaging with the trial but also the collective (i.e., the wider community of ALS patients). Through enhancing patient involvement in its "patient communities" and promoting observational trials like the lithium carbonate one, PLM then champions participatory practices where users are fully informed of the platform's functionality while never playing the role of paying consumer, as instead it happens on 23andme.

There are, however, two additional—and somehow intertwined—elements that need to be highlighted in PLM's overall business model: the "for profit" side of the platform and its "data openness". As Tempini (2015, p. 194) summarises: "because of how the data are controlled and the way the organization's business model is designed, most of the research [it] has produced has been dependent on the occasion of related commercial research projects". In fact, PLM finances itself through the sale of research services to "partners" (i.e., clients). These services are based on the data users generate on the platforms while engaging in self-tracking activities or socializing with other users the platform puts them in touch with based on shared characteristics (Tempini, 2015). In May 2021, PLM's website listed 71 "partners" classified as "non profit" (e.g., charities, advocacy organisations), "research and academia" (e.g., research centres, universities) or "industry" (e.g., pharmaceutical companies, health insurance plans) (PLM, 2021). The income produced by the sale of research services funds the continuous development of the digital platform as a knowledge sharing system, data aggregator and illness community enhancer and for the scientific research that the PLM company itself carries out and publishes (e.g., Wicks et al., 2010).

Compared to that used in the for-profit business model adopted by 23andme, the "gift exchange" between PLM and its users can probably be seen as more transparent. On the one hand, consumers can access the platform for free to journalise their everyday experience of health and illness, to be recommended and put in touch with other users and to access a number of report pages that provide snapshots about specific medical entities—namely, "symptom pages, treatment pages, and condition pages, all reporting various descriptive statistics" (Tempini, 2015, p. 197). On the other hand, they are clearly informed of their data being aggregated and sold, with an updated list of clients being clearly provided on the company's website. It is PLM's claims about its "data openness" that perhaps raise more questions. On its website, the company describes its mission as the following:

> PatientsLikeMe enables you to effect a sea change in the healthcare system. We believe that the Internet can democratize patient data and accelerate research like never before. Furthermore, we believe data belongs to you the patient to share with other patients, caregivers, physicians, researchers, pharmaceutical and medical device companies, and anyone else that can help make patients' lives better.
>
> (PLM, 2021)

However, in the context of PLM, data are only "open" to partners who pay to access them, a condition that hardly meets the criteria traditionally used to define "open data" in relation to access, redistribution and reuse (Kitchin, 2014, pp. 49–52).

The Infrastructural Drive of Corporate Tech Giants

In March 2015, researchers from Sage Bionetworks and the Center for Human Experimental Therapeutics and the University of Rochester Medical Center launched the non-profit health sector enterprise Parkinson mPower (PmP). PmP is an iPhone-based app used to monitor and track symptoms of Parkinson disease (Bot et al., 2016). The app was developed using Apple's ResearchKit library, another non-profit enterprise that allows researchers to gather (iPhone) user data in the form of survey responses, reports, physical measurements and assessments (Van Dijck & Poell, 2016, p. 7) The idea behind PmP is that via a large patient enrolment and the daily tracking of symptom data—both ensured by the use of a freely available mobile app—new and known patterns of Parkinson symptoms could be quantified and analysed.

The integration of the interconnected PmP, ResearchKit, and iHealthKit—a general health data storage service—in the Apple ecosystem, however, has a number of important implications for individuals' participatory potential and for the public good. First, only iPhone users can access PmP, resulting in a selected demographic being able to share their data and to be included in any study developed for the benefit of Parkinson patients. Thus, compared to PLM, PmP is an exclusive platform, in the sense that a large number of individuals, namely non-iPhone users, are excluded from it. Second, Apple has obvious control over the data flowing in its (proprietary) ecosystem of apps, with the potential to link large datasets generated and stored not only via PmP, ResearchKit, and iHealthKit but also via other apps in the ecosystem. This translates in "endless opportunities to combine and reuse stored databases" (Van Dijck & Poell, 2016, p. 8), with huge economic potential and, again, in a data system that can hardly be defined as open. Third, PmP's dependence on the Apple ecosystem points to the increasing infrastructural role of giant corporate actors. With the infrastructural turn of digital platforms (Plantin et al., 2018), major corporate entities (e.g., Apple, Google) have become increasingly essential to our daily lives: while controlling central hubs of the overall digital ecosystem, they dominate services of broad public value within profit-driven corporate models. On the one hand, this infrastructural turn causes the exclusionary environment that we mentioned earlier (Williams et al., 2020). On the other, it makes digital health platforms, as sectoral entities, embedded in an interconnected "global digital infrastructure—a structure on which many companies and states depend to build their platforms and online services" (Van Dijck, 2020, p. 5). As is clearly the case for PmP, the integration of non-profit digital health platforms within corporate ecosystems of apps allows data streams to flow seamlessly. The dependence on proprietary systems, however, effectively channels data, originally shared in a non-profit context, into a proprietary data flow often controlled by one corporation (e.g., Apple)'s platforms.

Nudging Engagement, Shaping Ephemeral Citizenship?

Founded in 2005, Care Opinion is a non-profit organisation offering a feedback website that uses a similar design to that of commercial ranking platforms (Petrakaki et al., 2021, p. 3). Originally based in the UK (Sheffield and Stirling), Care Opinion now has branches in Ireland and Australia. On careopinion.org, anybody can share feedback about specific health and care service providers (e.g., hospitals, GPs). This feedback is moderated by a team from within the organisation and redirected through the platform to referents from the said service providers. These referents are then invited to respond. The platform is designed in a way that "Everyone can see how and where services are listening and changing in response" (Care Opinion, 2021). In May 2021, the platform had collected 450,173 feedback stories, had 9,877 health and care staff subscribed to "listen" to these stories and had received a response for 77% of the stories received in the previous month (Care Opinion, 2021).

Care Opinion is somehow extremely different from the examples of digital health platforms examined in the previous sections because it is a non-profit organisation primarily funded through subscriptions from health and care service organisations. In other words, neither do data collected through the platform become an element of financial transactions (e.g., 23andme; PLM), nor do they enter the data flows of the wider digital ecosystem (e.g., PmP). In fact, when social science research started discussing the commodification of patient data through digital health platforms, Care Opinion would be used as a yardstick for comparison. For instance, Lupton (2014b, p. 866) would write:

> What is the nature of the digital assemblages . . . configured via interaction with a platform such as PatientsLikeMe compared with those produced by interacting with Patient Opinion,[1] for example? What kinds of value, commercial or affective, do these assemblages produce and attract? What are their politics?

As anticipated in Lupton's remarks, research on Care Opinion has since drawn attention to the "digital assemblages" forming on its platform, that is, it has shed light on the way users engage and interact with technologies embedded in it, resulting in new forms of knowledge practices, sociality and, potentially, participatory dynamics (see Ruppert et al., 2013). In particular, Petrakaki and colleagues (2021, p. 2) have analysed Care Opinion to explore how digital health platforms may enact forms of "digital health citizenship", namely "an assemblage of discourses, technologies and practices at the intersection of biosociality and "technosociality". Drawing from Novas and Rose (2000)'s conceptualisation of "biological citizenship" (see Chapter 3), Petrakaki and colleagues picture "digital health citizenship" as happening through the use of digital health platforms and as defined by—and itself defining—what it means to be active members of the community, with regards to individual and collective health choices. Their focus is very much on the way technological "nudges", in the form of, for instance, prompts, metrics, or recommendation systems, while motivating patients to engage on the platforms, produce "communities" that are algorithmically defined and, as such, not necessarily long-term expressions of citizenship. We can perhaps see this as another aspect of the fluidity that we described in Chapters 5 and 6 when discussing the forms of engagements enhanced by mainstream social media—Twitter in particular—in non-dedicated and non-binding digital environments.

Care Opinion also clearly exemplifies how engagement with digital health platforms does not necessarily translate into agency concretising beyond the platforms themselves: "Despite the best of intentions, demands for change raised in feedback platforms remain structured by their digital environment and are not embedded in the wider healthcare environment. As a result, patients' feedback might not necessarily be properly addressed" (Petrakaki et al., 2021, p. 7). In fact, patient stories posted on Care Opinion have been shown to generate a variety of reactions from health and care service providers, ranging from "non-responses, generic responses, appreciative responses, offline responses and transparent, conversational responses" (Ramsey et al., 2019, p. 42). Responses also vary in the extent to which they are specific to the patient story, transparent and suggesting ameliorative action planned to improve future care delivery. Interestingly enough, and seemingly corroborating Petrakaki et al.'s (2021) conclusions on the limited agency enacted by digital health platforms, Ramsey and colleagues' (2019) work shows that while transparent and conversational responses are those most likely to be desired by patients, they are actually those least likely to happen on Care Opinion.

Digital Health Platforms as Sociocultural and Material Artifacts

So far, in this chapter we have discussed some of the key implications of the political economy of contemporary digital health platforms for the development of participatory practices and new or renewed cultures of health and illness. In the present and the following sections, we will shift the focus to the way users engage with and potentially shape digital health platforms. This will require seeing and understanding platforms as sociocultural and material artifacts (Lupton, 2014a) rather than technological agents (e.g., Petrakaki et al., 2021), with the aim of building a fine-grained understanding of the way agency emerges and develops through technological engagement situated in everyday use practices. The following sections will focus on three core aspects of mundane, lived experiences of digital health: the affective dimension of health data, the attribution of meaning and values to platforms and data, and the labour exerted by platform users in repairing, curating and discerning data produced, stored and represented via platforms.

Feeling and Sensing Data on and Via Platforms

In their work on everyday experiences of data, Kennedy and Hill argue for the importance of understanding "the feeling of numbers", namely, how "data are as much felt as they are experienced cognitively and rationally" (2018, p. 831). They highlight how understanding data as rational entities translates into excluding the wide range of non-rational experiences—and all those who have those experiences—from theorisations of datafication.

While Kennedy and Hill (2018) point to a scarcity of sociological work interested in understanding emotions in the context of data and data visualisations, it is perhaps unsurprising that emotions and affective work have been at the centre of social science research focused on digital health platforms for some time now. As a matter of fact, health is a personal, social, and emotional aspect of our everyday life. In her (2014) pivotal work on personal analytics, Ruckenstein discusses how the very design of digital health platforms is based on the goal of making bodily information visible and urging individuals to check this information against internalised understandings of what is good and right. This process of "self-optimisation" is inherently affective because it is inspired by the desire of reaching an optimal self. On the one hand, it can work in a context where this optimal self is inspired by a notion of a healthy self constructed against rational and normative standards, often set by the platform itself (Fotopoulou & O'Riordan, 2017). On the other hand, it might prompt actions aimed at bypassing this normative "healthy" to pursue one's own notions of what is good and right, like in pro-ana communities (Ruckenstein, 2014, p. 71). This affective dimension is often enhanced by data visualisation practices where "visible outcomes, graphs and illustrations are critical for making the practice emotionally compelling" (Pantzar & Ruckenstein, 2015, p. 103).

To understand the emotional and sensory aspects of everyday engagements with digital health platforms, Lupton (2017b) suggests applying the notion of "affective atmospheres". This was coined within the field of cultural geography to address the feelings that characterise interactions—of both humans and non-humans—in specific places and spaces, as "perceived and felt through the body" (Lupton, 2017b, p. 1). The concept of affective atmosphere is especially attuned to interpret practices of care because these practices often involve emotional experiences related to understanding and living through health and illness. In the context of digital health platform use, humans "encounter" devices, often in very intimate ways (e.g., wearables), with these devices entering an almost symbiotic relationship with their users and populating affective atmospheres. These atmospheres are fluid: they form with the users' body and bodily data but constantly also incorporate data from other users (e.g., in groups or social activities). The sensory aspects of these interactions are evident both when platforms work well, for instance generating a positive emotional response (e.g., sense of achievement) and when they do not work, causing negative emotions (e.g., annoyance) (Lupton, 2017b, p. 5).

In sum, work on the affective dimension of platform experiences offers an understanding of data as contingent, contextual, processual, open, and relational rather than rational and cognitive (Sumartojo et al., 2016). This approach allows us to explore how data generated via digital health platforms are used to understand our own selves and imagine futures in ways that may or may not be aligned with those expected by platform providers and inscribed in platform "biopedagogies" (Fotopoulou & O'Riordan, 2017). In other words, by exploring how data are felt (Kennedy & Hill, 2018) and sensed (Lupton, 2017c), we can provide insight into the agentic work of users who tinker with digital health platforms to accommodate their own experiential understandings of health and illness.

The Meanings of Data in Everyday Life

If we acknowledge that everyday experiences of digital health platforms are marked by affective dynamics (Lupton, 2017b), we also hint at a relational aspect in users' understandings of data and data practices. Data can be seen as relevant based on very different value systems and this becomes evident from "the way different people talk about what they want from data and how they expect data to perform socially, organizationally, and institutionally" (Fiore-Gartland & Neff, 2015, p. 1478). Fiore-Gartland and Neff use the notion of "data valence" to explore the way different individuals, stakeholders and communities of practice see data as valuable. Their work provides evidence of six core valences being attributed to digital health data by different individuals among clinicians, technology designers and users: self-evidence, actionability, connection, transparency, truthiness and discovery. These valences may overlap and are not necessarily representative of a specific community of practice but show how data can be understood as valuable based on very different expectations of use. In their study, individuals expected data to be inherently right (self-evidence), to prompt corrective action (actionability) or conversations (connection), to be open and shareable (transparency), to be rational and objective (truthiness) or to act as means to explore and learn (discovery).

Drawing on Fiore-Gartland and Neff's (2015) terminology, we can add that a "data valence" often foregrounded by self-trackers, especially those engaging with the quantified self rationale, is that of self-awareness (Lupton, 2019). What is arguably most interesting here is that this self-awareness is searched for through "soft resistances" whereby platform users "dismantle the categories that make traditional aggregations appear authoritative" (Nafus & Sherman, 2014, p. 1785), like those informed by Foucauldian interpretations of biopower. In their study of the Quantified Self movement, Nafus and Sherman (2014, p. 1793) describe self-trackers' experimentations with tracking devices as still rooted in the logics and frameworks set by corporate platform providers—hence why their being "soft" forms of resistance that do not entirely escape "the wider biopolitics of late capitalism". These experimentations are however also exercises of tinkering or "wrestling" with given forms of both (algorithmic) data aggregations and constructs of health. Sharon and Zandbergen (2017, p. 1699) distinguish between three forms of "soft resistance" or, as they put it, "three other forms of meaning-making" that are used by members of the Quantified Self movement and probably apply to self-trackers more widely. Not only does these users' work dismantle views of self-tracking as a form of "data fetishism" grounded in understandings of data as inherently objective, rational and true; it also uncovers three alternative "data valences" (Fiore-Gartland & Neff, 2015). The first sees self-tracking as a practice of mindfulness, in which affective experiences are possible and desirable. The second values it as a way to resist social norms and conventions. The third frames it as a communicative practice, where data are used to share experiences across groups and types of expertise.

In sum, digital health platforms, as sociocultural artifacts, are spaces and places where users exert agency via constructing their meanings of and practices with personal and socialised health data.

Repairing, Curating, and Discerning Data

Acknowledging an affective dimension of platform and data practices, and one embedded in personalised interpretations of what data mean and why they matter, implies accepting that data, especially health data, are "lively" entities (Lupton, 2017d). Not only do health data concern the human body and its functions; they also travel across devices, users and use purposes and are subjected to algorithmic aggregations and filtering that ultimately have implications for the lives of individuals and social groups. As Lupton puts it, digital health data "are *dynamic assemblages* of humans and nonhumans that are constantly subject to change" (2018, p. 9, emphasis added). The coming together of these assemblages has a strong material component, one that becomes evident with the mundane, everyday engagement with the platforms (e.g., wearables) through which data are generated, visualised, shared, processed and/or stored. In fact, scholars interested in everyday uses of digital technology have drawn attention to the socio-materiality of data and platforms. Digital data have been described as having "forensic materiality", meaning that their formulation requires manipulating physical matter (e.g., a hard drive), and "formal materiality" in the sense that they are based on computational processes (Tanweer et al., 2016, p. 737).

Focusing on the materiality of digital health data allows us to explore instances in which matter, whether forensic or formal, breaks. The relevance of this opportunity lies in the fact that it is in these very instances that the relationships underpinning human-non-human assemblages in digital health practices become evident and "felt". That is to say, when platforms break or pause, and/or data halt, their users necessarily acknowledge their presence because they are urged to intervene and, possibly, engage in "repair work" that has agentic potential (Schwennesen, 2019). As Pink and colleagues put it: "a focus on breakage, repair and growth is an opportunity to learn about everyday data worlds, and to account for how these disrupt and break the linear, solutionist, and triumphant stories of Big Data" (2018, p. 11). In reflecting on his ethnographic investigation of the use of algorithmic systems in the context of health care, Schwennesen, for instance, highlights how "repair work" done by patients and health professionals in response to unexpected—and felt-wrong—technological response, is indicative of the need to see algorithmic systems—and data flowing through them—as fluid, situated in use contexts, and embedded in sociotechnical assemblages, rather than as monolithic, raw entities. Ultimately, this suggests that algorithmic systems are actually "open-ended" and interventions should be thought of how to further enhance means for users to respond to them, e.g., repairing, domesticating, adapting and fully appropriating them.

Building on the notion of "repair work", Weiner and colleagues (2020) extend the focus to the "curational work" done by individuals engaged in self-monitoring practices for health purposes, namely practices of filtering and only drawing attention to a selected pool of measurements. According to their study, it is not always completeness that self-trackers seek to achieve when tinkering with data and materials, it is rather accomplishment according to personal goals or expectations. As the authors put it:

> *discerning work* in the context of self-monitoring provides a broader term for describing the work that people do to create self-monitoring records . . . Here, data may be partial, but not necessarily broken, in the sense of representing an incomplete set of the data created and capturing the selectivity or interestedness of the data recorded.
>
> (Weiner et al., 2020, p. 12, emphasis added)

Ultimately, the pool of research discussed in this section identifies a range of activities through which platforms are domesticated by users, in instances of agentic work that participate in mundane digital health practices.

Conclusion: Eight Propositions on Digital Health Platforms and Participatory Cultures of Health and Illness

The global proliferation of digital contact tracing apps during the Covid-19 pandemic (see Ada Lovelace Institute, 2020) can be seen as emblematic of the way digital health platforms are increasingly relevant to individual users, social groups, health care services and society overall, with a knock-on effect on participatory practices in the management of health and illness. In this chapter, we have discussed both the challenges embedded in contemporary neoliberal political economies and technological systems and the opportunities emerging in everyday sociocultural and material user practices. Ultimately, the chapter suggests that digital health platforms relate to contemporary cultures of health and illness by hindering or channelling participation. We can summarise this through the following propositions:

1. **Health and patient data collected via digital health platforms are likely to be commodified: once on the platform, they enter financial transactions that in most cases exclude their original owners—the individuals whose personal information is being transacted and monetised.** These

individuals often receive compensation in the form of self-satisfaction for engaging with what is framed as altruistic action—or participation in research. In practice, this "participation" primarily translates into waiving personal data ownership, leaving little space for other forms of agency or decision-making regarding what is being researched and how. Not only does this align with a view of patients and laypeople in general as "auxiliary" (see Chapter 3); it also opens up new space for commercial entities to shape health and care decision-making.

2. **Digital health platforms are dataveillance systems: their very functioning is grounded in objective understandings of health and illness meant to quantify and monitor own selves and others through platform-driven and often market-driven norms**. Through the use of these platforms, users become experts of their bodies. This expertise, differently to that we discussed in Chapter 3, is however at least partially shaped by what is deemed measurable and valuable by the platforms themselves, which also set the standards against which body values must be assessed.
3. **Data flowing within and across digital health platforms are often addressed as "open" but, in reality, they are hardly so if their access is limited and only available to few "partners" or "clients', like in for-profit contexts.** Data are simply "not open" when they are not equally accessible to everyone.
4. **Digital platforms are increasingly becoming essential to our daily life, with this infrastructural turn seeing major corporate entities (e.g., Apple, Google) working as hubs of the overall digital ecosystem and dominating services of public value through profit-driven corporate models**. This makes for digital health platforms embedded in a global digital infrastructure that also often integrate non-profit digital health platforms within corporate ecosystems. Data originally shared in a non-profit context is then often channelled into proprietary data flows controlled by one corporation, a solution hardly conducive to the development of alternative or bottom-up participatory initiatives.
5. **The citizenship developing on digital health platforms is at least partially defined by technological "nudges", in the form of, for instance, prompts, metrics, or recommendation systems that, while motivating patients to engage on the platforms, produce "communities" that are algorithmically defined and, as such, not necessarily long-term expressions of citizenship**. Hence the question: can these forms of citizenship still have long-term effects and produce change?
6. **Despite working in dataist and market-driven contexts, digital health platforms are experienced and domesticated by their users, who exert agency by tinkering with their own data, measurements, and contacts.** This tinkering represents a new dimension in the thriving of the experiential understandings of health and illness that we discussed in Chapter 3 and can be the basis for the formation of new or renewed epistemic communities populated by laypeople.

7. **Data mean different things to different people, and as such they can also become a means for resistance.** This resistance is "soft", in its being shaped by the dataveillance environment discussed earlier, but may constitute a form of participatory drive carved in a now almost entirely market-driven system.
8. **Domestication and soft resistance develop via the individual and social curation, repair and discerning of data produced, collected and/or stored via digital health platforms.** Platform users have purposes and agendas that fit with their life and, sometimes, with the life of their illness subculture. These purposes and agendas shape uses and practices in ways that often resist norms dictated by market, biopolitical or technicist systems.

Note

1. Care Opinion was formerly named "Patient Opinion'.

Reference List

23andme (2021). 23andme.com.

Ada Lovelace Institute (2020, July 9). *COVID-19 digital contact tracing tracker*. www.adalovelaceinstitute.org/project/covid-19-digital-contact-tracing-tracker/

Bot, B. M., Suver, C., Neto, E. C., Kellen, M., Klein, A., Bare, C., . . . Trister, A. D. (2016). The mPower study, Parkinson disease mobile data collected using ResearchKit. *Scientific Data*, *3*(1), 1–9.

Byer Shainman, A. (2019). Amy Byer Shainman. *FORCE*. https://www.facingourrisk.org/get-involved/how-to-help/volunteer-fundraise/volunteer-spotlight/amy-byer-shainman.php

Care Opinion (2021). www.careopinion.org.uk/

Charitsis, V. (2019). Survival of the (data) fit: Self-surveillance, corporate wellness, and the platformization of healthcare. *Surveillance & Society*, *17*(1/2), 139–144.

Charmaz, K. (1991). *Good days, bad days: The self in chronic illness and time*. Rutgers University Press.

Esmonde, K., & Jette, S. (2020). Assembling the "Fitbit subject": A foucauldian-socio materialist examination of social class, gender and self-surveillance on Fitbit community message boards. *Health*, *24*(3), 299–314.

Fiore-Gartland, B., & Neff, G. (2015). Communication, mediation, and the expectations of data: Data valences across health and wellness communities. *International Journal of Communication*, *9*, 19.

Fotopoulou, A. (2018). From networked to quantified self: Self-tracking and the moral economy of data sharing. In Papacharissi, Z. (Ed.) *A networked self: Platforms, stories, connections* (pp. 144–159). Routledge.

Fotopoulou, A., & O'Riordan, K. (2017). Training to self-care: Fitness tracking, biopedagogy and the healthy consumer. *Health Sociology Review*, *26*(1), 54–68.

Foucault, M. (2019). *Ethics: Subjectivity and truth: Essential works of Michel Foucault 1954–1984*. Penguin UK.

Gillespie, T. (2010). The politics of "platforms". *New Media & Society*, *12*(3), 347–364.

Hands, J. (2013). Introduction: Politics, power and "platformativity". *Culture Machine*, 14.

Harris, A., Wyatt, S., & Kelly, S. E. (2013). The gift of spit (And the obligation to return it) how consumers of online genetic testing services participate in research. *Information, Communication & Society*, *16*(2), 236–257.

IDC (2020, December 2). Shipments of wearable devices leap to 125 million units, up 35.1% in the third quarter, according to IDC. *IDC*. www.idc.com/getdoc.jsp?containerId=prUS47067820

Jewell, T. (2020a, August 12). The best fitness and exercise apps of 2020. *Healthline*. www.healthline.com/health/fitness-exercise/top-iphone-android-apps#map-my-run

Jewell, T. (2020b, August 12). The best healthy lifestyle apps of 2020. *Healthline*. www.healthline.com/health/mental-health/top-healthy-lifestyle-iphone-android-apps

Kallinikos, J., & Tempini, N. (2014). Patient data as medical facts: Social media practices as a foundation for medical knowledge creation. *Information Systems Research*, *25*(4), 817–833.

Kennedy, H., & Hill, R. L. (2018). The feeling of numbers: Emotions in everyday engagements with data and their visualisation. *Sociology*, *52*(4), 830–848.

Kitchin, R. (2014). *The data revolution: Big data, open data, data infrastructures and their consequences*. Sage.

Langlois, G., Elmer, G., McKelvey, F., & Devereaux, Z. (2009). Networked publics: The double articulation of code and politics on Facebook. *Canadian Journal of Communication*, *34*(3).

Lupton, D. (2014a). Apps as artefacts: Towards a critical perspective on mobile health and medical apps. *Societies*, *4*, 606–622.

Lupton, D. (2014b). The commodification of patient opinion: The digital patient experience economy in the age of big data. *Sociology of Health & Illness*, *36*(6), 856–869.

Lupton, D. (2016). The diverse domains of quantified selves: Self-tracking modes and dataveillance. *Economy and Society*, *45*(1), 101–122.

Lupton, D. (2017a). *Digitised health, medicine and risk*. Routledge.

Lupton, D. (2017b). How does health feel? Towards research on the affective atmospheres of digital health. *Digital Health*, *3*, 2055207617701276.

Lupton, D. (2017c). Feeling your data: Touch and making sense of personal digital data. *New Media & Society*, *19*(10), 1599–1614.

Lupton, D. (2017d). Lively data, social fitness and biovalue: The intersections of health self-tracking and social media. In Burgess, J., Marwick, A., & Poell, T. (Eds.) *The SAGE handbook of social media*. Sage.

Lupton, D. (2018). How do data come to matter? Living and becoming with personal data. *Big Data & Society*, *5*(2), 2053951718786314.

Lupton, D. (2019). "It's made me a lot more aware": A new materialist analysis of health self-tracking. *Media International Australia*, *171*(1), 66–79.

Marwick, A. (2012). The public domain: Surveillance in everyday life. *Surveillance & Society*, *9*(4), 378–393.

The Medical Futurist (2019). Feeling sick? There's an app for that! *The Big Symptom Checker Review*. https://medicalfuturist.com/the-big-symptom-checker-review/

Nafus, D., & Sherman, J. (2014). Big data, big questions| this one does not go up to 11: The quantified self movement as an alternative big data practice. *International Journal of Communication*, *8*, 11.

Novas, C., & Rose, N. (2000). Genetic risk and the birth of the somatic individual. *Economy and Society*, *29*(4), 485–513.

Pantzar, M., & Ruckenstein, M. (2015). The heart of everyday analytics: Emotional, material and practical extensions in self-tracking market. *Consumption Markets & Culture*, *18*(1), 92–109.

Petrakaki, D., Hilberg, E., & Waring, J. (2021). The cultivation of digital health citizenship. *Social Science & Medicine*, *270*, 113675.

Pink, S., Ruckenstein, M., Willim, R., & Duque, M. (2018). Broken data: Conceptualising data in an emerging world. *Big Data & Society*, *5*(1), 2053951717753228.

Plantin, J. C., Lagoze, C., Edwards, P. N., & Sandvig, C. (2018). Infrastructure studies meet platform studies in the age of Google and Facebook. *New Media & Society*, *20*(1), 293–310.

PLM (2021). *Partners*. www.patientslikeme.com/about/partners

Quantified Self (2021). *What is quantified self?* https://quantifiedself.com/

Ramsey, L. P., Sheard, Dr, L., & O'Hara, Dr, J. (2019). How do healthcare staff respond to patient experience feedback online? A typology of responses published on Care Opinion. *Patient Experience Journal*, *6*(2), 42–50.

Ruckenstein, M. (2014). Visualized and interacted life: Personal analytics and engagements with data doubles. *Societies*, *4*(1), 68–84.

Ruppert, E., Law, J., & Savage, M. (2013). Reassembling social science methods: The challenge of digital devices. *Theory, Culture & Society*, *30*(4), 22–46.

Saukko, P. (2018). Digital health: A new medical cosmology? The case of 23andMe online genetic testing platform. *Sociology of health & illness*, *40*(8), 1312–1326.

Schüll, N. D. (2018). Self in the loop: Bits, patterns, and pathways in the quantified self. In Papacharissi, Z. (Ed.) *A networked self and human augmentics, artificial intelligence, sentience* (pp. 25–38). Routledge.

Schwennesen, N. (2019). Algorithmic assemblages of care: Imaginaries, epistemologies and repair work. *Sociology of Health & Illness*, *41*, 176–192.

Sharon, T., & Zandbergen, D. (2017). From data fetishism to quantifying selves: Self-tracking practices and the other values of data. *New Media & Society*, *19*(11), 1695–1709.

Sumartojo, S., Pink, S., Lupton, D., & LaBond, C. H. (2016). The affective intensities of datafied space. *Emotion, Space and Society*, *21*, 33–40.

Tanweer, A., Fiore-Gartland, B., & Aragon, C. (2016). Impediment to insight to innovation: Understanding data assemblages through the breakdown: Repair process. *Information, Communication & Society*, *19*(6), 736–752.

Tempini, N. (2015). Governing PatientsLikeMe: Information production and research through an open, distributed, and data-based social media network. *The Information Society*, *31*(2), 193–211.

Tutton, R. (2002). Gift relationships in genetics research. *Science as Culture*, *11*(4), 523–542.

Van Dijck, J. (2014). Datafication, dataism and dataveillance: Big Data between scientific paradigm and ideology. *Surveillance & Society*, *12*(2), 197–208.

Van Dijck, J. (2020). Seeing the forest for the trees: Visualizing platformization and its governance. *New Media & Society*, 1461444820940293.

Van Dijck, J., & Poell, T. (2016). Understanding the promises and premises of online health platforms. *Big Data & Society*, *3*(1), 2053951716654173.

Weinberg, J. (2020). Are symptom tracker apps the future of healthcare? Is the use of symptom tracker apps set to explode in a post-pandemic world? *Raconteur*. www.raconteur.net/healthcare/symptom-tracker-apps/

Weiner, K., Will, C., Henwood, F., & Williams, R. (2020). Everyday curation? Attending to data, records and record keeping in the practices of self-monitoring. *Big Data & Society*, *7*(1), 2053951720918275.

Wicks, P., Massagli, M., Frost, J., Brownstein, C., Okun, S., Vaughan, T., . . . Heywood, J. (2010). Sharing health data for better outcomes on PatientsLikeMe. *Journal of Medical Internet Research*, *12*(2), e19.

Wicks, P., Vaughan, T. E., Massagli, M. P., & Heywood, J. (2011). Accelerated clinical discovery using self-reported patient data collected online and a patient-matching algorithm. *Nature Biotechnology*, *29*(5), 411–414.

Williams, R., Will, C., Weiner, K., & Henwood, F. (2020). Navigating standards, encouraging interconnections: Infrastructuring digital health platforms. *Information, Communication & Society*, *23*(8), 1170–1186.

World Health Organization and International Telecommunication Union (2020). *Digital health platform handbook: Building a digital information infrastructure (infostructure) for health.* Licence: CC BY-NC-SA 3.0 IGO. https://apps.who.int/iris/bitstream/handle/10665/337449/9789240013728-eng.pdf

8 Conclusion

Understanding Participatory Cultures of Health and Illness in Contemporary Societies

Introduction

The extent to which the digital has come to shape both everyday life and societal systems has gradually also transformed our approaches to knowing society. Social science research is now increasingly searching for strategies that develop a "beyond the media" focus to capture digital transformations happening across many societal sectors. In fact, the interface between media and wider architectures has also emerged in several chapters of this book (see, in particular, Chapters 2, 4 and 7).

It is extremely important to bear in mind that we live in "digital" (Marres, 2017) or "platform" (Van Dijck et al., 2018) societies that are characterised by distinct—though often intersecting—cultural, social, and political dynamics. This book mainly draws upon Western examples and scholarly work, so the society explored here is primarily a Western one. I am hoping, however, that at least some of the considerations drawn in the course of the previous chapters and brought together in the points below might talk to dynamics beyond the West and/or inform future comparative research into participatory cultures of health and illness across societies.

In the last two chapters, I advanced a series of propositions to understand how contemporary digital platforms enhance or hinder participatory cultures of health and illness. These propositions have both methodological and conceptual dimensions and should be seen as potentially informing future research on how we live, experience and construct meanings and practices around health and illness on and through digital platforms. In this concluding chapter, I draw on these considerations, reflect on the questions raised at the end of the pandemic snapshots presented in Chapter 1, and ultimately delineate five key aspects that should inform future research into participatory cultures of health and illness. The five points presented below respectively focus on 1) digital participation as connective, personalised and crowdsourced agency, 2) the media side of digital participation, 3) lay expertise as a digital participatory practice, 4) the corporate gateways of digital participation, and, finally, 5) digital participation as platformed.

DOI: 10.4324/9780429469145-11

1. Digital Participation as Connective, Personalised and Crowdsourced Agency

In conversation with Mizuko Ito and Danah Boyd, Henry Jenkins reminds us that:

> Many of the debates of our time center around the terms of our participation: whether meaningful participation can occur under corporately controlled circumstances, when our ability to create and share content is divorced from our capacity to participate in the governance of the platforms through which that content circulates.
>
> (2016, p. 12)

It comes with no doubt that the "politics of platforms" (Gillespie, 2010) limits users'—and produsers'—agency (see Chapter 2). Guo Jing's snapshot (see Chapter 1) provides clear evidence that these constraints work across platform ecosystems, whether these are predominantly shaped by state (e.g., China) or free market (e.g., West) capitalist values (see, for instance, Vicari and Yang, forthcoming). Our everyday engagement with digital platforms turns into traces that live at the intersection of the private and the public, get translated into data easily transferable across platforms' gateways (i.e., APIs,) and acquire economic value that primarily benefits platform corporations (Van Dijck et al., 2018). And yet, citizen participation still surfaces through online deliberative practices (Jackson et al., 2020), data activism (Milan & Van der Velden, 2016), and digital citizenship (Hintz et al., 2018). But how does this happen when deliberations, data and citizenship have to do with health and illness?

In Chapter 5 we saw that traditional, patient-driven, health advocacy actors increasingly rely on digital mechanisms that enhance the co-production of health knowledge and offer individualised routes of public engagement with issues related to health and illness. Participation here translates into agency that is connective, personalised and crowdsourced (Bennett & Segerberg, 2013) and that often sees lay people, especially patients and carers, finding themselves and each other in fluid illness subcultures fed by varied (e.g., traditional, alternative, credentialed, experiential) information pathways. These encounters may lead to the emergence of publics—and counterpublics—in more or less fluid spaces on mainstream social media platforms, where experiential and expert knowledge often intersect, producing extensive epistemic work (see Chapter 6).

This connective, personalised and crowdsourced agency also surfaces in data-driven forms of participation—and citizenship (e.g., Petersen et al., 2019; Petrakaki et al., 2021)—on digital health platforms. Not only do they emerge in explicit and intended acts of resistance (e.g., Nafus & Sherman, 2014); they also occur in the mundane digital (Pink et al., 2017). In Chapter 7 we saw that users here experience and domesticate platforms by tinkering with their own data, measurements, and contacts. This tinkering develops via repair work (Pink et al., 2018), individual and social curation, and data discerning activities (Weiner et al., 2020) and ultimately shapes uses and practices in ways that often resist norms dictated by market, biopolitical or technicist systems.

2. The Media Side of Digital Participation

When the slogan "Don't hate the media, be the media", became indie and pop at the end of the 1990s (see Chapter 2), there was perhaps an expectation that Indymedia's bottom-up, alternative and possibly radical model of media content production would last, or become more mainstream.

Contemporary media systems—as intertwined with wider digital infrastructures—are indeed far from monolithic or, for instance, reducible to Western or "Global North" models (Chan, 2013; Milan & Treré, 2019). Most forms of participation, especially deliberation, happening online in contemporary societies are however strongly influenced by both old and new "media logics" (Altheide & Snow, 1979): they often focus on legacy media coverage—which is based on traditional news value systems—and develop on "new" (i.e., digital) media infrastructures—which allow bottom-up and crowdsourced content production while being primarily controlled by profit-driven giant corporations (see Chapter 2). The hybrid dimension (Chadwick, 2017) that emerges at the intersection of these logics is then simultaneously influenced by the values and norms characterising legacy media content production and by the values, norms *and affordances* characterising digital media platform ecosystems. Needless to say, this dimension is very different from that inscribed in the participatory model iconised by the 1990s "be the media" part of Indymedia's manifesto and, before that, by the view of the Internet as a "free gift to the community" (Curran & Seaton, 2010, p. 263). In fact, as seen at point 1, contemporary hybrid media logics are conducive to participation that is often highly influenced—and constrained—by capitalist structures. Point 4 below will further explore this by discussing the platform side of these logics.

3. Lay Expertise as a Digital Participatory Practice

The idea that experiential knowledge can be as valuable as professional knowledge dates back to at least the 1970s (e.g., Borkman, 1976) and became a key angle to understand the "lay expertise" developing within health advocacy groups in the 1990s (Epstein, 1995) (see Chapter 3). In fact, debates about "experiential knowledge" and "lay expertise" have drawn increasing attention to the way lay knowledge and expertise related to health and illness can lead to forms of "proto-professionalism" (Caron-Flinterman, 2005, p. 2577). On the one hand, experience has proven key to understanding a dimension of disease that has become increasingly important also in clinical settings: its lived aspects. On the other hand, a tension to familiarise oneself with professional knowledge has turned evident across patient groups, especially in relation to conditions about which information is limited and/or hardly accessible, giving way to forms of citizenship that have been defined as "biological" (Rose & Novas, 2005) (see Chapter 3).

In sum, the 1990s progressive shift in the understanding of patienthood as an active form of engagement with health conditions, and the increasing relevance of lay expertise to citizenship practices, have provided a fertile background for the proliferation of personalised forms of engagement and knowledge co-production that came into being with the turning mundane of social media practices. Digital socio-technical infrastructures have probably accelerated and enhanced the *public* or *semi-public* manifestation of these pre-existing or emerging participatory dynamics in what have become "bio-digital" forms of citizenship (Petersen et al., 2019). It is then probably due to this combination of non-platform bound sociocultural dynamics and platform-specific socio-technical infrastructures that the public voice of collective advocacy actors and individual patient advocates has progressively grown in prominence.

As seen in Chapter 6, on mainstream social media platforms "lay experts" can easily become exemplars within illness subcultures and/or gatekeepers of scientific information. When it comes to digital health platforms (see Chapter 7), lay expertise, as a digital participatory practice, is cultivated and retrained through data and data work, with a constant tension between biopolitical forces—e.g., "biopedagogies" (Fotopoulou & O'Riordan, 2017)—and personalised data curation practices.

4. Digital Participation Through—or Despite—Corporate Gateways (Aka, the Usual Foes)

In one way or another, all points above take us back to the political economic forces that drive contemporary societies. Whether we look for agency carved within market, biopolitical or technicist systems (point 1), explore the media side of contemporary digital participation (point 2) or investigate the evolution of lay expertise as a digital participatory practice (point 3), we always end up having to account for the "(overwhelmingly corporate) global online platform ecosystem that is driven by algorithms and fueled by data" (Van Dijck et al., 2018, p. 4).

As seen in Chapter 7, while becoming central to our daily life, digital platforms have undergone a process of infrastructuralisation (Plantin et al., 2018), with major corporate entities (e.g., Apple, Google) becoming hubs of the overall digital ecosystem and dominating services of public value through profit-driven corporate models. This makes digital media embedded in a global infrastructure that often integrates non-profit digital platforms within corporate ecosystems.

Platform companies' handling of the personal data collected, stored and/or shared on digital platforms often turns lay people into data donors, with the alleged goal to "advance research". When it comes to data donated in the context of patient groups, the process often turns patients into "auxiliary" to research, annihilating most of the participatory agency achieved by patient advocacy groups in the 1990s and early 2000s (see Chapter 3). In other words, this turns "active patients" back into "data donors". Meanwhile, the transactions characterising these data handlings open up new space for commercial entities to shape health and care decision-making. In fact, digital health platforms often work as "dataveillance systems" Lupton (2016)—grounded in rational and objective understandings of health and illness dictated by market-driven norms. In these systems, data are then often commodified entities and hardly "open": their access is restricted to platforms' "partners" or "clients". Even data originally shared in a non-profit context are then often channelled into proprietary data flows controlled by one corporation. This scenario may allow soft forms of resistance (Nafus & Sherman, 2014) but excludes more radical, alternative, or bottom-up participatory initiatives from the mainstream.

5. Digital Participation as Platformed

Together, the points above suggest that digital participation is now overwhelmingly platformed in both its agentic constraints and potential. Constraints to agency cannot but emerge in an ecosystem whose very essence is defined by contemporary platform politics: these politics are shaped by capitalist values driven by the giant corporations that act as infrastructural hubs; they function through algorithmic norms that define what (e.g., content, users) should or should not be visible; they shape social interactions via affective vernaculars voiced through platform markers (e.g., emojis). Digital participation, as platformed, is however also allowing and enhancing connective, personalised and crowdsourced forms of agency that are inclusive of fluid and loose instances of participation, and that were rarely possible in the pre-digital age.

When it comes to participatory cultures of health and illness, these dynamics translate in a context hardly conducive to quick systemic changes or radical projects. A context that, however, opens up opportunities for illness subcultures to grow, especially around minorities (e.g., rare disease or non-communicable disease communities) whose members have little opportunities to find each other "offline". It also translates in forms of "togetherness" that can take a myriad of shapes, as digital connective structures also offer means of engagement for individuals unwilling or unable to strongly commit to traditional advocacy or activist action. Finally, it manifests itself in the heightened visibility of lay forms of expertise that previously only primarily grew within contained or dedicated—thus often "invisible"—social spaces.

Reference List

Altheide, D. L., & Snow, R. P. (1979). *Media logic*. Sage.

Bennett, W. L., & Segerberg, A. (2013). *The logic of connective action: Digital media and the personalization of contentious politics*. Cambridge University Press.

Borkman, T. (1976). Experiential knowledge: A new concipept for the analysis of self-help groups. *Social Service Review*, *50*(3), 445–456.

Caron-Flinterman, J. F., Broerse, J. E. W., & Bunders, J. F. G. (2005). The experiential knowledge of patients: A new resource for biomedical research? *Social Science & Medicine*, *60*, 2575–2584.

Chadwick, A. (2017). *The hybrid media system: Politics and power*. Oxford University Press.

Chan, A. (2013). *Networking peripheries: Technological futures and the myth of digital universalism*. MIT Press.

Curran, J., & Seaton, J. (2010). *Power without responsibility* (7th ed.). Routledge.

Epstein, S. (1995). The construction of lay expertise: AIDS activism and the forging of credibility in the reform of clinical trials. *Science, Technology & Human Values, 20*(4), 408–437.

Fotopoulou, A., & O'Riordan, K. (2017). Training to self-care: Fitness tracking, biopedagogy and the healthy consumer. *Health Sociology Review, 26*(1), 54–68.

Gillespie, T. (2010). The politics of "platforms". *New Media & Society, 12*(3), 347–364.

Hintz, A., Dencik, L., & Wahl-Jorgensen, K. (2018). *Digital citizenship in a datafied society*. John Wiley & Sons.

Jackson, S., Bailey, M., & Welles, B. (2020). *#Hashtagactivism: Networks of race and gender justice*. MIT Press.

Jenkins, H., Ito, M., & boyd, d. (2016). *Participatory culture in a networked era: A conversation on youth, learning, commerce, and politics*. John Wiley & Sons.

Lupton, D. (2016). The diverse domains of quantified selves: Self-tracking modes and dataveillance. *Economy and Society, 45*(1), 101–122.

Marres, N. (2017). *Digital sociology: The reinvention of social research*. John Wiley & Sons.

Milan, S., & Treré, E. (2019). Big data from the South (s): Beyond data universalism. *Television & New Media, 20*(4), 319–335.

Milan, S., & Van der Velden, L. (2016). The alternative epistemologies of data activism. *Digital Culture & Society, 2*(2), 57–74.

Nafus, D., & Sherman, J. (2014). Big data, big questions| this one does not go up to 11: The quantified self movement as an alternative big data practice. *International Journal of Communication, 8*, 11.

Petersen, A., Schermuly, A. C., & Anderson, A. (2019). The shifting politics of patient activism: From bio-sociality to bio-digital citizenship. *Health, 23*(4), 478–494.

Petrakaki, D., Hilberg, E., & Waring, J. (2021). The cultivation of digital health citizenship. *Social Science & Medicine, 270*, 113675.

Pink, S., Ruckenstein, M., Willim, R., & Duque, M. (2018). Broken data: Conceptualising data in an emerging world. *Big Data & Society, 5*(1), 2053951717753228.

Pink, S., Sumartojo, S., Lupton, D., & Heyes La Bond, C. (2017). Mundane data: The routines, contingencies and accomplishments of digital living. *Big Data & Society, 4*(1), 2053951717700924.

Plantin, J. C., Lagoze, C., Edwards, P. N., & Sandvig, C. (2018). Infrastructure studies meet platform studies in the age of Google and Facebook. *New Media & Society, 20*(1), 293–310.

Rose, N., & Novas, C. (2005). Biological citizenship. In Ong, A. & Collier, S. (Eds.) *Global assemblages: Technology, politics and ethics as anthropological problems* (pp. 439–463). Blackwell Publishing.

Van Dijck, J., Poell, T., & De Waal, M. (2018). *The platform society: Public values in a connective world.* Oxford University Press.

Vicari, S., & Yang, Z. (forthcoming). Humans, Covid-19 and platform societies in *Being Human during Covid-19*.

Weiner, K., Will, C., Henwood, F., & Williams, R. (2020). Everyday curation? Attending to data, records and record keeping in the practices of self-monitoring. *Big Data & Society, 7*(1), 2053951720918275.

Index

Note: Page numbers in **bold** indicate tables.

23andme 135–136, 140, 142

Acquired Immune Deficiency Syndrome (AIDS) 42, 46, 48–49
active patient 41, 46, 70, 126, 156
Ada Lovelace Institute 5, 147
affective public 29
agency: beyond produsage 21–22; civic 24–25, 31; community 81; individual 88, 91, 138, 143; levels of 109; organisation's 80; patients' 39, 66, 69, 91, 139; rhetorical 30; structures of 65, 94; user 146–149
Akrich, M. 69–70, 112, 121, 127
American Civil Liberties Union (ACLU) 103–104
Angelina effect 101, 125–126
Application Programming Interface (API) 6, 22, 24, 154
autism 42

Battle of Seattle 16
Batt-Rawden, Samantha 6
Bennett, Lance: on crowdsourcing agency 154; on curation 101; on digital mechanisms 76; on the logic of connective action 86–87, 92–93, 104, 107, 109, 125; on personal life stories 23, 26–28
bio-digital citizenship 75
biographical disruption 43, 66, 79, 112
biological citizenship 50, 142
biopedagogy 138
biopower 138, 145
boundary movement 40, 48, 51–52, 81
boundary object 52
BRCA: content curation 101–107; epistemics 119–124; frames 107–112; genetic mutations 101; storytelling 112–119
breast cancer: activism 38, 44; blogs 66–67; genetic risk 101–103, 107, 109; self-advocacy 46, 105; themes 111, 125
Breast Cancer Action (BCA) 102–103, 109
broadcaster 28, 102–107
Brown, Phil 38–40, 48, 51–53, 82, 92–93
Bury, Michael 43–46, 66, 79, 112

Care Opinion 134–135, 142–143
Chamak, Brigitte 40–42, 46, 48
Charmaz, Kathy 43–44, 139
citizen journalism 20
clicktivism 21
community of practice 69, 119, 120, 145
connective action: in the BRCA Twitter stream 104–109, 125; the logic of 25, 76–77; on rare disease organisation websites 92, 94
contact tracing 5–6, 147
context collapse 122
counterculture 17, 28
counterpublic 25, 28–29, 32, 154
curation: dynamics 125, 126–127; in self-monitoring 147, 149, 154, 156; of social media content 28, 100–107, 111

data activism 23–24
datafication 22–23, 31, 144
dataveillance 137–138, 148–149, 157
digital activism 15, 154

digital citizenship 23, 75, 154
digital health 61, 119, 133, 143, 145–146
digital health platform 64, **90**, 119, 133; and participatory cultures 147–150; the political economy of 135–143; as sociocultural and material artefact 143–147
digital mechanism 28, 76, 86–89, 99, 154
digital medicine 61

eHealth 61, 63
embodied movement 40, 48, 53
emoji 7, 113, 115, 118, 127
epatient 61, 65–69, 71
epistemic community 70, 119–121, 148
Epstein, Steven 8, 38–42, 48–49, 75, 155
European Medicine Agency (EMA) 76, 94
European Organisation for Rare Diseases (Eurordis) 51, 53
experiential knowledge: and boundary movements 52; concept of 38, 47–49; and dataism 138; in epistemic communities 121; and experiential information 69–70; and lay expertise 155; patients' 84, 93–94; publics' 89

Facebook: data 65; feeds 22, 87–88; group or pages 92–93, 100; as platform 20, 31, **90**, 99, 119; post 123; as source **106**, **110**
Facing Hereditary Cancer Empowered (FORCE) 103
Fitbit 134–138
Food and Drug Administration (FDA) 76, 90, 94
frame 29–30, 107–111

gatekeeper: and broadcaster 102–106; of expert information 123, 126, 128, 156; Twitter 29
genetic testing 49–50, 93, 101, 104, 121
Global Justice Movement 15–16

Hardey, Michael 66, 69–70, 112, 116, 126
hashtag activism 29–30
health activism 39–42
health advocacy: and activism 39–42, 53, 75; digital 92, 100; organisations 104, 154; and rare diseases 51, 86
health social movement 39–40, 41, 44–45

illness identity 42–44, 92
illness narrative 44–46, 53, 66, 112
Indymedia 16
influencer 29, 102, 115, 126
Instagram 31, 99–100, 113, 116, 122
interconnectivity 93
International Telecommunication Union (ITU) 133
intraconnectivity 92
issue public: ad hoc 29; and epistemics 119–121; and hashtag activism 30; health 125–128; on social media 25–26, 28, 107

Jing, Guo 1–2, 23, 154
Jolie, Angelina 101–102, 105–112, 125

lay expert: activists 48–49; exemplars of gatekeepers 128, 138, 156; in support groups 51, 69
lay expertise: as a digital participatory practice 153, 155–156; and experiential knowledge 38, 47–51, 138; and knowledge production 69; and storytelling 116
Long Covid 3–5
Lupton Deborah: on dataveillance systems 157; on digital health platforms 119; on experience economy 135–137; on health and social media 99; on platforms as artefacts 142–146; on self-tracking citizenship 139; on wearables 61, 63–64, 66

Mallendar, Louise 122–123, 128
meme 30–32
mHealth 61, 63–64
Murphy, Lesley 113, 115–116

National Organization for Rare Diseases (NORD) 51, 53, 91
networked counterpublic 29
networked public 92
networked sociality 18
new genetics 49–51
Novas, Carlos 46, 50–51, 75, 142, 156

open data 135, 141
Open-Source Movement 19
Orgad, Shani 45, 66, 68–69, 112–113, 115, 126
Orphan Drug Act 51, 79, 83

Papacharissi, Zizi: on the commercialisation of platforms 67; on networked framing 107, 109; on personalised activism 76; on social media and democratisation 24–25; on social media content curation 27–31, 125; on Twitter as news reporting mechanism 127; on Twitter as storytelling medium 112
Parkinson mPower 141
participation 8
participatory culture 8, 99–158
participatory practice: and data activism 23; digital 16, 22; and digital health platforms 147, 153, 155–156; and health knowledge 91–92; and lay expertise 51; mundane 94; and platform politics 32, 54, 135, 140, 143; and public engagement 76; and shared illness 44
patient advocacy: digital mechanisms for 86–91; evidence of **124**; groups 156; organisations 40–42, 48, 53, 75, 79, 82; rare disease 78, 80
patient advocacy organisation 40–43, 48, 53, 79, 82
PatientsLikeMe 134, 138–142
Perego, Elisa 3–5
Petersen, Alan 8, 50–51, 76, 154–156
platformisation 22–23, 102
produsage 15–21
produser 17–21, 154
public sphere 24–25, 29, 32

Quantified Self movement 137, 145

Rabeharisoa, Volovona 42, 50–52, 75, 77, 80, 82–83
Rabinow, Paul 76
rare disease 46, 51–53, 75–94, 104, 157
resilient issue public 119–120
Rose, Nikolas 46, 50–51, 75, 142, 156

self-advocacy 46–47, 53
selfie 31, 99
slacktivism 21
spreadability 31
storytelling: approach 66; and illness narratives 45; and sources of information 121–123, 126, 127; Twitter 101, 112–119
surveillance 17, 63–65, 70, 136–138

telemedicine 61–64
TikTok 99
Twitter 31, 65, 87–88, 90, 92–93, 100–128

user-generated content (UGC) 19–21

Van Dijck, Jose 19–22, 135–138, 141, 153–154, 156
virtual community 16–17

WeChat 1, 11
Whole Earth 'Lectronic Link (WELL) 17
Wikipedia 20
World Health Organisation (WHO) 90

For Product Safety Concerns and Information please contact our EU
representative GPSR@taylorandfrancis.com
Taylor & Francis Verlag GmbH, Kaufingerstraße 24, 80331 München, Germany

www.ingramcontent.com/pod-product-compliance
Ingram Content Group UK Ltd.
Pitfield, Milton Keynes, MK11 3LW, UK
UKHW021447080625
459435UK00012B/400

* 9 7 8 1 0 3 2 1 6 9 5 8 3 *